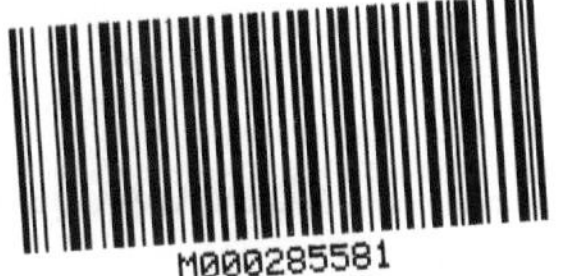

Praise for

'Dr Bhaswati has written a book that will help resurrect the knowledge I grew up on, using scientific logic for modern scientists, and slokas for ancient scientists and observers. Her writing will appeal to the intelligent seeker dedicated to achieving a good life using conscious self-care, attention to healthy habits and respect for the wisdom of the ancients.'

Shashi Tharoor,
member of Parliament

'Bhaswati combines her talents as a healer with passion for sharing truly healing medicine. She has written from the song in her heart that celebrates light, sound and connection with nature.'

Pandits Rajan and Sajan Misra,
Padma Bhushan recipients and classical
Hindustani vocalists of the Banaras Gharana

'Bhaswati is uniquely able to diagnose like good medical doctors of the past, watching the patient rather than the test result. With a person-centered approach, this book is a tribute to Āyurveda and explains why we should pay more attention to the signals our bodies give us.'

Ashok H. Advani,
founder publisher, The Business India Group

'Bhaswati has preserved the Sanskrit from which *dinacharya* emanates. Through her unending curiosity and dedication as a well-trained physician, scientist and professor, she has brought basic concepts of Āyurveda to light. She has toiled and delved deeply with engaging clarity, a fine mind and an extraordinarily connected soul. She teaches Āyurveda authentically because it is in her heart.'

Dr Vd. Chandrabhushan Jha,
former dean, faculty of Āyurveda, Banaras Hindu University and professor emeritus of Rasa Shastra

'Ancient Āyurvedic rishis developed *dinacharya*, a way of maintaining normal body rhythms and staying healthy. Assisted by logic and personal accounts, Dr Bhaswati brings *dinacharya* alive in this book and reinforces its importance and necessity, especially in busy lives.'

Vd. Partap Chauhan,
founder of Jiva Ayurveda

'Dr Bhaswati unlocks the age-old tenets of Āyurveda contained in cryptic Sanskrit verses. Her strong roots in tradition and willingness to branch out to the modern world make this book precious, like any true vidya.'

Dr P.R. Krishnakumar,
Padma Shree recipient and managing director,
Arya Vaidya Pharmacy, Coimbatore

'As a fellow Fulbright Scholar, I have witnessed Dr Bhaswati devote her life to researching and preserving Āyurveda, and bringing it back to the hands and hearts of people.'

Gautam Gandhi,
former head of new business development, Google India

Everyday Āyurveda

Everyday Āyurveda

Daily Habits That Can Change Your Life

DR BHASWATI BHATTACHARYA

Foreword by Abhay Deol

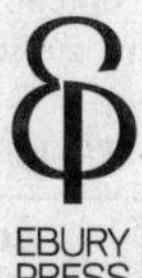

EBURY PRESS

An imprint of Penguin Random House

EBURY PRESS

USA | Canada | UK | Ireland | Australia
New Zealand | India | South Africa | China

Ebury Press is part of the Penguin Random House group of companies whose addresses can be found at global.penguinrandomhouse.com

Published by Penguin Random House India Pvt. Ltd.
4th Floor, Capital Tower 1, MG Road,
Gurugram 122 002, Haryana, India

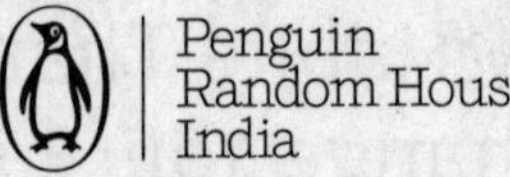

First published by Random House India 2015

18 17

ISBN 9788184004571

The views and opinions expressed in this book are the author's own and the facts are as reported by her which have been verified to the extent possible, and the publishers are not in any way liable for the same.

For sale in the Indian Subcontinent only

Typeset in Times New Roman by Manipal Digital Systems, Manipal

Printed at Replika Press Pvt. Ltd, India

www.penguin.co.in

To the three men
to whom I made promises
from my soul

For devotion, KB
For discipline, PBM
For daring, BCB

Foreword

My whole life, I have believed in Āyurveda. To use its principles in a practical way and to mould it to a crazy schedule like mine is what I have always sought. It is what many of us seek but do not find in easy, accessible ways.

Bhaswati does exactly that. She makes Āyurveda practical while also preserving its authenticity. Her logic and stories, with her impressive background as a well-qualified medical doctor, scientist and public health specialist from some of the best schools (Harvard, UPenn, Columbia, Princeton, Rush, Cornell and BHU) make the book that much more valuable. Since I have met her in New York, Bhaswati has made it her mission to bring the wisdom of Āyurveda back to the people in a usable, everyday way.

As an eco-environmentalist and a thinking actor, I often explore good food and sound health choices to keep my skin and face healthy and my body fit, and consume a diet that both satisfies and nourishes.

Āyurveda rejects the stale, easy, ready-in-a-minute choices in the urban world of jets, trains and film sets, and encourages all things natural. Through this ideology, I have learnt how to understand what my body needs and make choices that allow me to do fun things and still be healthy.

Getting up early is one thing that feels really good. Though I often have late-night engagements that require sleeping in, I am finding that *Brahma muhurta*—rising with the sun—actually helps keep my body strong.

When Bhaswati first told me about *gandusha* for teeth whitening, I enthusiastically asked to learn how to partake! What a great thing to hear the logic and her explanation on how to do it. I offered to be the face for her remedies.

Bhaswati is the person who has taken Āyurveda from ancient wisdom and brought it into the modern day. When people ask her how a modern medical doctor can be so supportive of Āyurveda, she gives a cannonball of evidence.

She is smart, she is articulate, and she is kind. Her clinical practice is her best evidence. Her treatments and approaches integrate the best of authentic Āyurveda, which we know and love, with the practical needs of modern medicine.

When she told me about her book, I was extremely happy. Instead of chasing her down with each skin problem, I now have a handbook to guide me through a strong regimen. She can slightly alter most of the treatment in the book to my particular *dosha* to make it a medical treatment.

This is also a fun book to read. The writing is unapologetically sensual and spiritual, and reveals her own encounters since childhood amid nature and the ways of Āyurveda. It will benefit those who want to make and see changes in their health.

Abhay Deol

Preface

Many moons ago, my mornings began in the usual modern, urban Western way: waking up to an alarm clock, a cup of coffee, a quick shower and a whirlwind of multitasking that included checking emails and patient lab reports, eating while organizing the apartment and packing my briefcase before rushing to a metro ride to the hospital. I was efficient, accomplished and pleased.

After a few years, when I began gaining weight, my hair became dry and began to fall, and my gut was bloated too often, I thought these were the inevitable symptoms of aging. A voice deep inside questioned how some people were healthy even in their eighties, while others got sick. Modern medicine had few answers, but lots of tests and drugs to suppress those inescapable symptoms.

Thus, I was provoked onto a journey of questioning whether depletion is unavoidable. I delved deeper into Āyurveda and found a road introducing me to the concepts of *dinacharya* (daily routine). Once I succumbed to that inner voice, I became more curious and more aware of many things. I consciously veered away from the usual path and chose to open a quiet solo private practice, wary to enter the limelight of celebrity physicians who tend to become blinded about their primary roles as healers.

Through the many *grantha*s, or great scriptures, I learnt that from the time of the Vedas—around 10,000 BCE—until 500 CE, wise men continuously used, perfected and refined the knowledge of life, longevity and well-being, known as the *veda* of *ayus*, or Āyurveda. This knowledge was hidden over the past 200 years, in the most nefarious conquest India faced: the conquest over self-awareness.

But as I began to revisit India more regularly, I found that the wisdom still existed, in pockets and quiet corners of the country, handed down quietly from generation to generation, as traditions of healing and wholeness, known sometimes as Āyurveda and sometimes simply as tradition. They need no validation or approval; their observations and healthy patients are enough.

When I first started practising Āyurveda, I was told it was preventive, and that the best way to engage was with single herbs, some yoga poses, and some diet and lifestyle changes. Done authentically and aligned with the philosophical concepts of Āyurvedic *dosha*, *guna*, *agni* and *srotas*, my prescriptions began to include a section for lifestyle counselling specific to the patient. I began to prescribe fewer drugs, surgeries and tests, and more herbs, oils, routines and yoga asanas. Slowly, my practice transformed to include what I learnt from patients and old, wise physicians, what I read in medical journals and ancient texts, and what I gleaned from my heart.

Holistic medicine became my work and my play, as I witnessed healing of conditions that were impossible to cure with my black bag of modern medicine. I checked tests and scans, patients told me their stories and I began to believe. In 2003, one of the community hospitals of Cornell Medical College opened a holistic women's health clinic in New York that I directed for years until I moved into full-time private practice. My students requested that a small institute experimenting with holistic medicine be integrated into their modern medical training. Only after opening The DINacharya Institute did I begin to explore the power of our namesake more deeply.

What I have found is what I want to share with you: my journey of discovering lifestyle interventions, such as scraping the tongue and oil massages before bathing, are not only preventive, but are actually curative interventions that will heal and rejuvenate you. This collection contains forty-two sections from the granthas of Āyurveda, offered with logic, practical hints, some science and some stories.

This book is written for the person who has unwittingly accepted influences of urban culture, subliminal messages in television ads and conventional medicine's approach to health, science and truth. Popular culture disseminates the general philosophy that we should consume more, have more, buy more and do more without considering the impact on ourselves, our families, our communities and our planet. As part of the movement of adopting sustainability, holistic medicine and natural approaches to health and wellness, an understanding is emerging among those committed to awareness. Ancient practices may seem rustic and outdated, but they are as relevant now—after we see what our consumerism is doing to the planet—as they were 100 years ago. If we can return to being connected to the land, we can heal conditions we thought incurable.

What we need is not to be younger, but to be revitalized, resilient, reconnected with our hearts and re-energized to journey through the learning that is life. *Dinacharya* restores our *agni*, or inner fire, unclogs our senses, strengthens our mind and connects us to our soul, empowering us to transform our lives.

❧

Prologue

Moist soil peeks through my little toes as I sit on my mother's lap, gazing at the passing countryside as we whirl past in a rickshaw. The same air that kissed nearby shrubs swirls gently on to us as my mother tells my mashi (aunt) about medicinal salves and potions made from the neem tree. Mashi listens only somewhat intently, watching the mélange of hues in this lush tropical Bengal countryside that is my ancestral land. Thick underbrush occasionally jumps out on to the road as we rush to the train station on an overcast afternoon. Each time my five-year-old arms unleash into the wind, my mother instinctively pulls me closer to her silk smoky blue-grey sari as the cool monsoon humidity caresses my shoulders and wraps around us. The rustic smell of soil touches our soul, a refreshing change from the thick hot city air and the previous weeks of summer. My mother pays no apparent attention to the rickshaw wallah, but is aware of his presence and our complete dependence on him to transport us safely.

This is the forest of my childhood, where I still go to play. This is where I breathe deep, fearless breaths of lustful life, unapologetically sensuous and daringly spiritual. Among these trees, wisdom is fresh and knowledge is deep. Each day presents new colours and sounds that exemplify their strangely familiar and stable dependence on routines that make sense of the world.

Part I:
Early Morning Rituals

Waking from that lush neem forest into the dimness of the predawn hour and my father's familiar stride past my oak door, I enter the reality of my large corner bedroom in this expansive old brick house. The wooden boards creak in familiar places as I rise, chanting to my feet for the past two decades in this powder-blue room.

It is just before dawn. My father, as usual, has descended from his bedroom and uses his cane and coordination to hobble down a flight of stairs to the kitchen. My sleepy-eyed countenance satisfies him. '*Chaa*,' he states and goes to his chair in the dining alcove. He and I are both grateful that this routine is known to both of us. In my half-awakened daze, I instinctively make him black Darjeeling tea, taking care to steep the leaves to the proper mahogany colour in his favourite English cup. Half-filled cardboard boxes lie dozing all over the kitchen, reminding me that I have to come to terms with the fact that we are moving out of the very house in which my father had hoped to die.

Over the next half hour, I talk as my father actively nods, bright-eyed from the tea's sweep over his somnolence. He is verbally silent since his stroke five years ago, but his presence is thunderous.

❧

Part I:
Early Morning Rituals

~ • 1 • ~

Rise and Shine

When I was a young girl, my father would wake me. '*Oatt. Oatt.* Get up . . .!' Babi—our *dak naam* (nickname) for my father—would burst into our room before the crack of dawn, igniting the room with an energy that tousled with our dreams. '*Ghummocho? Ghummocho*? Are you sleeping?' He would come in and sit on the bed near my feet, and bounce, '*Uttecheesh? Uttecheesh?* Are you awake yet?'

'No, Babi.'

'Then *oatt.* Get up. It is the hour of Brahma! "Early to bed and early to rise makes a good girl healthy, wealthy and wise." *Oatt. Oatt.*' In our house, parents are second only to God. When parents command, children do not argue. I would rouse myself reluctantly, leaving the softness of my sister's arms, and stamp out, groaning, to meet him in one of the main rooms. My father wanted me to make the most of these sacred, early-morning moments. He would chant mantras until I had no resolve but to waken and join him.

Sometimes we would sit. Sometimes we would stroll around the veranda as he sipped the tea made for him. If the weather permitted, we would go walking to take in the fresh oxygen that the trees had started brewing for us at the light of dawn. When we returned to the warmth of the house, my father would sit on the floor and chant sacred mantras that awaken the brain. Sometimes he would talk to me about his topic of the day, usually something to do with the sperm that swam through the years of his career as a spermatologist and infertility specialist, or later, his work on HIV and immunology.

Once, at the age of eleven, he had given me a *Scientific American* article extolling the immense brain capacity of children before puberty. Following suit, he began waking me at 4 a.m. for weeks to have me recite the-R groups of all twenty amino acids. Aliphatic: glycine–H, alanine–methyl or CH_3; branched chain: valine–ethyl, leucine–ethyl-dimethyl, isoleucine–methyl-isopropyl . . . Then he had forced me to read Lehninger's *Biochemistry* cover to cover to understand his work better. I did not understand most of the words or structures or what they implied about the mechanisms of the body. Nonetheless, it was required reading. Somehow, it was easy in those early hours. I could memorize anything then.

❧

That is how I learnt about *Brahma muhurta*. The period from 4 a.m. to 6 a.m. is sacred to Brahmins. To all who are acquainted with Āyurveda, these are the hours of *vāta*, when lightness of being is present, when the soul can most easily be accessed by our heavy, thick material minds. *Brahma muhurta* is literally translated in Sanskrit as the moments (*muhurta*) of *Brahma*, the energy of the creator, as the day is created consciously in the moments just before dawn.

brahme muhurte uttisthet swastho raksartham ayushah: |*1*|

To preserve a wholesome life of health and protect his wisdom and happiness, one should rise early during the period of Brahma muhurta.

Astānga Hrdaya of Vāgbhata,
Sūtra-sthāna; chapter 2, sloka 1

Ideally, we should rise between 4 a.m. and 6 a.m., depending on the latitude and time zone in which we live. We should spend 1–2 hours with ourselves before the world demands our time of us. Sages knew this. Farmers knew this. They knew they needed to maximize the time in their fields during the light of day. They used this predawn time to get their bodies and minds ready so that the remainder of the day could be spent outside.

Āyurveda teaches that these morning hours have a lightness of being. They should be spent in that space between mind and body, where our spirit attunes us most easily to our life purpose. It is the most fresh and pure time of day, and provides the cleanest oxygen for exercise and for connecting with the purest part of our selves. Those who want to ride the wave of lightness, clarity and subtle energies may meditate or go for a euphoric morning run. Follow your instinct and watch your body's reaction; adjust according to how it worked for you. This self-adjustment through trial and error, and observation is called *upasaya*, advised by Āyurveda as one of the best ways of tailoring what you need for your body.

- Rise early, between 4 and 6 a.m.
- Spend 1–2 hours with yourself.
- Meditate or go for a morning run to imbibe lightness, clarity and subtle energies.
- Follow your instinct on which activities work for you by gauging your body's reaction.

According to generations of ancient wise men, who were a combination of astrophysicist, geologist and expert biologist, the day is composed of thirty periods of 48 minutes each, called *muhurtas*. *Brahma muhurta* is two periods before dawn, in the span during twilight. If sunrise occurs at 6 a.m., *Brahma muhurta* at that location on that day is from 4.24 a.m. to 5.12 a.m., changing daily.

The wise men used this time to expand their knowledge, as it symbolized light in all its meanings: illumination, wisdom, heat and buoyancy. It is the last part of the night, before the sun rises to proclaim a new day. The environment is also cleanest, containing the least pollutants, since people and animals sleep, as trees accelerate their production of clean oxygen using the white, pre-bright light of the sun. Noise and calls are absent from the predawn pleasant atmosphere of lightness, clarity and subtle energies.

This span of 96 minutes before dawn until 48 minutes before dawn is like prime time for sacred transmissions between the gods and our bodies.

There are many sacred ways to split the day into sections, such as the *prahāra* system of eight blocks of 3 hours. *Prahāras* are reference periods indicating when particular activities should take place. The first *prahāra* begins at sunrise and is for rising and meditation. The second *prahāra* is for starting the day, setting up the home and preparing morning food. Eating during this second *prahāra* is ideal for keeping digestive and immune systems healthy. The penultimate *prahāra* from midnight to 3 a.m. is the time for sleep. The last *prahāra* is the time just before dawn, for ending sleep, lovemaking and rising. This *ashtam prahāra*, or eighth and last *prahāra* of the daily cycle, extends from 3 a.m. to 6 a.m. and is used to guide musicians about which compositions are optimal at this time for maximum alignment with nature and the body.

Sometimes, these three-hour blocks are also called *yāmā*. (Note that this term is different from *yama*, which means restraints in yoga shastra.) Like *prahāra*, *yāmās* denote times of the day correlated with the power and angle of the sun, and optimal activities during these periods.

- The first *prahāra,* beginning at sunrise, is for rising and meditation.
- The second is for starting the day, tidying up the home and cooking the morning meal.
- The third *prahāra* is ideal for eating.
- Sleep during the penultimate *prahāra*.
- The last *prahāra*, the period just before dawn, is for lovemaking and rising.

According to Āyurveda, the early morning embodies the principle of *vāta*.

Vāta, *pitta* and *kapha* are the three *dosha*s of the body. *Dosha*s are principles of nature or forces that manifest from non-material energy, laced with the intentions of consciousness. They apply to everything on the planet and in the universe, as conceived by humans.

Āyurveda understood that all things move between energy and matter. The sophisticated system of philosophy called *sankhya* posits that all that is material is derived from energy and intentions of the *paraatma*, or universal soul. It presumes that all the play of the material world is simply a derivative of the soul's attempt to journey. This purposeful journey requires slower speeds than the lightning speed of soul, much as our need to slow down the car when we are searching for a specific address. Therefore, the soul manifests into material form and is governed by these three forces of nature known as the *dosha*s. In modern Indian languages, the term *dosha* refers to areas of vulnerability or faults, implying that our energetic souls are vulnerable in physical form.

According to post-modern physics and particle physicists who study what space is made of, that space between the nucleus of an atom and the electrons that spin around it is filled by something that can be affected by intention, perhaps called . . . consciousness. 'Hard-core' scientists like to ignore these theories and the data that does not fit with their pre-hardened concepts of what is real, creating problems for the rest of us for the past 500 years. They have denied the reality of consciousness as an element of science, yet it has emerged in the field of physics, blooming between their hard-core doubts. Āyurveda incorporated this idea of consciousness in its original foundations by grounding our minds' intentions in these *dosha*s.

*Dosha*s are not physical entities, nor are they 'the elements'. They are principles or forces that reflect the qualities of the elements—ether/space, air, fire, water and earth. Air and ether/space are the lightest elements. They are light, cold, dry, rough and mobile. The theme underlying these qualities is movement. Both air and space are transparent and yet tangible through their movement and interactions with the physical world. We sense space through sound. We sense air through the wind and our ability to touch, as well as through sound.

In the body, the theme of movement occurs in a multitude of needed functions and the five associated structures that are needed to fulfil those functions.

Area of Focused *Vāta*	Movement
Lungs	Breathing
Vessels	Circulation of blood
Joints	Physical movement
Colon	Movement of wind in the gut
Brain and nerves	Nerve impulses

Diseases in these areas disturb the theme of movement and therefore, unbalance *vāta* in the body. They are called *vāta* diseases and healed by replacing turbulent flows, cacophony, eddies and hurricanes with gentle flow, silent winds and sound.

The body requires *vāta* to be present for all movement to happen. It is called the king of the *dosha*s because it is through movement that all things begin and progress.

In the mind, *vāta* is the reflection of the quality of movement. When the mind is light, cold, dry and mobile, the person has a *vāta* mind. In balance, the person is creative, a fast thinker, quick to solve problems and a visionary. When the person is out of balance, *vāta* manifests as anxiety, fear, mental worry and insomnia. Most psychiatric and psychological conditions have a *vāta* component.

Āyurvedic wise men looked at the patterns of movement that determined the behaviour of the physical universe, both influenced by invisible forces as well as by human conscious intentions. Modern theories are now discovering the importance of looking at these biological patterns throughout the universe, instead of simply defining diseases based on what is seen anatomically in the body.

Explaining disease by incorporating the forces underlying biology, chemistry and physics, scientists have started looking at 'automatic' behaviour and what determines it. Functional connectomics of neurons studies how and why brain cells connect and flow to create brain function. Swarm intelligence looks at mass behaviour of one unit, such as bees, using intelligent flow patterns. Cluster epidemiology looks at how disease spreads between individuals and communities. Cymatics looks at the echo-type effects that sound and vibration have on solids and liquids in predictable patterns. In Āyurveda, all of these flows and patterns were called *vāta* as they were ruled by microscopic and macroscopic forces that specified movement.

The morning *vāta* brings lightness, clarity, coolness and a subtle energy into the body and mind. People with a light, lithe body who have a balanced sense of lightness and clarity can achieve ethereal heights during this time. They love to imbibe the *vāta* qualities in nature that match their own *vāta* abundance in their bodies and use the high for the rest of the day. People who have a heavier, stocky body can use the same wave of lightness to dislodge their inertia and move into an airy zone of being, since all beings have some *vāta*. But people who have both light, lithe bodies and heavy inertia-laden minds can actually mismanage their energies by starting movement or creative activities in a manner that is not smooth. Āyurveda uses meterology as an analogy; as light winds mix with heavy air, the imbalances in the air can produce tornadoes that extend from the atmosphere to the ground. These tornadoes can create mental havoc on *vāta* people or those with *vāta* disorders. It is better for them to do grounding activities, such as meditation or slow yoga. The ultimate balancer, if possible, is to spend time in nature.

Those people with extra weight or disorders of the body that produce unnatural heaviness, such as tumours, congestion and immune disorders, should be careful when bringing wind and lightness into the body, which is already heavy with confusion. This extra *vāta* energy can imbalance and provoke the body's imbalances further. The best option for these people is to wake and sit with a cup of sharp, awakening tisane (brewed spices in water without tea leaves) or tea if stimulation is needed. Meditation and time in nature are great equalizers for them too. A little later in the morning, they can engage in creative work and use the *vāta* energies to carry them into the *kapha* period of mid-morning.

If a person has a healthy mind and body, the early hours of *Brahma muhurta* quickly add healthy *vāta* to the body. Healthy *vāta* activities offset unhealthy *vāta* flows and dilute imbalances. For example, a person consumed by worry can shift that imbalance by rising early each morning and grounding the hyperactive, worried mind with a walk in nature or with a healthy, structured workout. Strenuous exercise, an unstructured morning of arguments or a scurry of activity will not ground the person. During these hours, a person can quickly replace the aberrant *vāta* flows with healthy *vāta* by engaging in the most spacious secure space, the mind. Therefore, no matter how tired a healthy person feels, the magic of the early morning should not be missed.

- ❧ People with light bodies and minds should make the best of the *vāta* period.
- ❧ Those with heavy, stocky bodies should use it to move into a lighter zone.
- ❧ People with light bodies but heavy minds should immerse themselves in grounding activities like meditation, slow yoga or spending time in nature.
- ❧ Do not bring in extra *vāta* if you have tumours, congestion and immune disorders. Drink hot tisane on awakening.
- ❧ The early hours of *Brahma muhurta* quickly add healthy *vāta* to the body if a person restores towards a healthy body and mind.

Āyurveda suggests we surrender to the awesome powers of nature that inherently rule us. It cycles from the macrocosm to the microcosm, stating, 'as in the world out there, so in the body in here'. There are three recurring cycles in nature, driven by forces that correspond to physiology in our body.

The first is the rotation of the earth on its axis, causing the day–night cycle. This is understood by the body through the pineal gland in the brain, found in many animals, which produces a series of chemicals, such as melatonin, and a cascade of signals along the hypothalamic–pituitary axis (HPA). These signal thoughts, emotions and activities via hormones, neurotransmitters and chemicals throughout the body that react in a fine-tuned web of intercommunication.

The second cycle corresponds to the revolution of the moon around the earth. This gravitational lunar pull produces cyclic tides of the ocean, due to the frictional coupling of water with the earth's rotation through the ocean floors, the inertia of water's movement, ocean basins that get shallower near land and oscillations between different ocean basins. It correlates to the menstrual cycle and corresponding hormonal flows in both men and women.

The third cycle corresponds to the revolution of the earth around the sun. It produces seasons and changes in nature that flow into cycles of perennial death and rebirth of flowering plants and herbs. The trees change their rhythms, as do animals, fields and water. We perceive these changes in the environment through our five senses and fires in our bodies, increasing our internal fires when the it is cold and decreasing them when it is hot.

These cycles and the principles of Āyurveda are not random. They correspond to a keen awareness of astrophysics and the ways in which the forces in the larger universe affect our bodies. To understand Āyurveda, we must remind ourselves continually of the adage, 'as in the macrocosm, so in the microcosm'.

There is evidence that the body attunes to the cycles of nature. In the deep of the night, just after our deepest sleep, around 4.30 a.m., our bodies are at their lowest body temperature. Low body temperatures are associated with healing, as proteins work slower and create less waste at low temperatures. Restorative functions take over, and build up and strengthening of tissues—healthy *kapha*—occurs during this time. Thus, we see that people living in colder climates tend to live longer, and sages tend to move up into the hills and higher altitudes. Each day, our body dips into this low temperature to give us a new start.

In preparation for rising, one of the body's most prominent protective hormones, cortisol, rises to its peak during the *vāta* period, around 6 a.m. Cortisol rises to help deal with the stress of waking up from a dormant body and disconnected mind. Attuning to cortisol, our stress hormone, through our conscious activities helps us rule our rhythms and rule our mind.

About 2 hours after *Brahma muhurta*, just after sunrise, we experience our sharpest rise in blood pressure, needed to help us become active for the day. This rise in blood pressure correlates with a sharp transient rise in adrenaline. It is well known that this increase of adrenaline and blood pressure is thought to be responsible for the statistic that most heart attacks occur during these early morning hours globally.

Around 7.30 a.m., melatonin secretion—which begins in the deep of the night—halts for the day. Melatonin rules the night as the precursor of serotonin, the mood-lifting brain chemical. Serotonin is at its highest level in the body early in the morning. Melatonin is one of the many chemicals produced in the brain by the pineal gland, which is sensitive to sunlight. It is part of a series of chemicals and cascade of signals along the hypothalamic–pituitary axis in the brain, coordinating the body through hormones, neurotransmitters and chemicals that interact throughout the body. When the coordination gets mangled, symptoms of imbalance arise.

Anyone who has worked the night shift knows the practical reality of not sleeping at night. Modern medicine finally validated the connection in the 1990s between functions of human physiology and the night–day cycle, called the circadian rhythm, and the field of chronobiology emerged. A series of accidents over recent decades by sleepwalkers, unrested resident physicians, night-time factory workers, nurses, young parents, truck drivers and pilots has increased research in chronobiology. Āyurveda tells us that misalignment with the hormonal cycles will plant seeds of imbalance that lead to mental and physical disease.

The theme of *vāta* is movement. The two *vāta* periods of the day span the movements and changes during sunrise and sunset, approximately 3–7, both in the morning and afternoon. These periods correspond to nature's ebbs and flows, and correlate with the daily rhythm of day and night, produced by the rotation of the earth on its axis.

Why were these early moments of the day so significant to the ancient people who marked them? The flows initiated during this period set the tone for the rest of the day. In the modern, urban lifestyle of today, 3–7 a.m. is still *vāta* time, ideal for three themes of activity—spirit, self and security. It is the time of renewal and reconnection with our inner strengths. From 4 to 6 a.m., we should ideally spend time in reflection, peace, nature, meditation, yoga and similar activities that unite the mind and spirit with the body and the life we have created. From 6 to 7 a.m., we should prepare for the coming busy stretch of morning.

- From 4–6 a.m., spend time in reflection, peace, nature, meditation, yoga and similar activities.
- Between 6 and 7 a.m., prepare for the day ahead.

Our rhythms are set early in life according to our routines, which are generally established by our parents and how we are brought up. To get back to the natural innate rhythm that all biological creatures have with the earth, a person should focus on good habits in the late evening and work towards good sleep that allows for early rising.

Of course, this is the biggest challenge of the modern, urban world. Society is simply not geared to reward healthy routines and rest at the end of the day. We struggle, attempting to juggle all the activities that are proposed to us in the evening hours. It is these evening hours that actually set the tone for the coming day. In the evening, a whole set of rituals is delineated by Āyurveda, known as *ratricharya*, or a wise nightly routine, addressed at the end of this book.

These rituals incorporate the evening tasks; how to adjust oneself if travelling, awareness of the environment conditions for the next half day, use of alcohol, engagement in sex, the evening meditation practice, conscious conclusion of the day with recall and review, and then the *rasayana* of sleep, or *nidra* yoga.

If the rituals of rest, nurture and care are met, the body, mind and senses re-find balance in space and time, and can become ready for the next round of life's journey. All too often though, the body remains exhausted, the mind remains agitated and the senses remain clogged. The next day is further exhausting, and the lessons and opportunities in front of a person are not seen.

These rituals are important because most of us are completely unaware of their potency in affecting our daily productivity.

To get started towards awareness, note mentally or on paper, your activities after sunset. Where do you go? What do you do? With whom do you spend time? Which kinds of activities engage your five senses? With whom do you share intimacy? The answers to these questions will reveal more to you about your day's outcomes than the activities in the light of day.

❧ Note down your activities after sunset: where you go, what you do, with whom you spend time, which kind of activities engage your five senses and with whom you are intimate.

Since Āyurveda is an individualized system, there are exceptions to every guideline. The rule of rising early does not apply to children under four, to the elderly, healthy or imbalanced, to parents with small children who are up at night and need to rest in the early morning and to people with illnesses or recovering from illness.

~ • 2 • ~

Old Food, New Food

As a child, I would often awaken early in the morning, just before my elders or sisters. Of course, my urge was to giggle and start playing, but I was usually scolded and told to lie silently and wait until my bedmates opened their eyes. Eventually, they would rise and spend some time in silence, eyes closed, just laying still. Then they would reach down and touch the floor. Only then was I allowed to move on the bed and commence play.

In college, when I began spending time with new roommates and friends, at sleepovers and camps, I noticed that none of them would awaken and spend time in silence before rising. It occurred to me that not everyone awakens into quiet time. No one would reach down to the floor. I then attributed my parents' silence to private prayers and never probed further. One day, decades later, my mother asked me whether I assessed my belly before I moved; whether I touched Mother Earth. I was blank.

❧

sharira-chintām nirvartya krtashauchavidhistatah: ||*1*||

With little or no movement, we should lie still and consider our belly.

Astānga Hrdaya of Vāgbhata,
Sūtra-sthāna; chapter 2, sloka 1

Āyurveda makes us conscious of our consciousness and our being in our body. It tells us to frame our world when we first awaken, before opening our eyes and moving mentally into the outside world, before getting out of bed. It asks us to connect consciously with our body. Start the day thinking of the source of your activity, your food.

During this time, we should consider the digestion status of the food eaten the previous day and night. Is the gut feeling clean? Is there pain? Is there hunger? Over time, this communication pathway strengthens with use, and one becomes more conscious of the gut. It is through this daily engagement that yogis learnt to develop control over their autonomic functions. On a subliminal level, knowing your hunger level and digestive strength may help you choose foods that are actually good for your system.

Āyurveda advises, 'you are what you digest' not 'you are what you eat'. Once you have started practising this second *dinacharya* ritual each morning, you will start to notice your feelings of satiety, anxiety, true hunger, queasiness, bloating, gas movement or calm.

If you overate, you probably digested a lot of excess and feel the excess; your body will have a dampened fire. If you drank yourself into a stupor before falling asleep, you probably digested a lot of stupor and astringency, and your body will have a dampened fire. This morning practice will start to increase your consciousness around your habits that may not be serving your body and soul.

After talking with your belly, move into a quick mental exercise to unite your mind and body. First sense the energy of the day with your non-visual senses. Spend a few moments connecting with the larger cosmos. Breathe through the top of your head directly into your heart space (the centre of your chest, not the physical heart). You can visualize a golden, luminous stream of compassion and love coming to you from all of your spiritual teachers, past, present and future, and from all realized beings. Feel a sense of grace expanding throughout your body. Rub your palms together quickly to generate warmth and then gently massage your face. Repeat this sequence for your head, arms and hands with long, smooth strokes.

When you have gently massaged your entire body, including your feet, sit on the edge of your bed facing north or east. Say a little prayer asking for help to act appropriately and grow, or simply expressing sincere gratitude for having found your dharma in this lifetime. If it feels real, you can generate a desire for the liberation of all beings and send that out.

- Lie silently and still for a few moments on waking.
- Evaluate the condition of your digestive system during this time.
- Visualize a quick mental exercise to unite the body and mind.
- Rub your palms to generate heat and gently massage your face. Repeat to deliver energy to all parts of your body.

❧

Before getting out of bed, reach down and touch the floor with your hand. Bend fully, gently and briefly. Āyurveda suggests that we touch the earth before walking all over her all day in an ode of respect. On a practical level, this bending compresses the abdomen and helps to move the old contents of the intestines down and out, a movement called *apana vayu*, to ready for excretion and cleansing of the body's main canal, called *srotoshodhana* (*srota* = channel; *shodhana* = cleanse).

Upon rising, Āyurveda suggests *ācamana*, that you drink a palmful of water from your right hand. The water should be either lukewarm or at room temperature, but not ice cold. Ideally, it should be boiled and stored overnight in a copper container. Copper is one of the necessary trace elements for the body, something people have forgotten from fear of heavy metals. The minuscule parts per million (ppm) of copper help to strengthen the muscles and cleanse the intestines.

This early morning water is said to stimulate the stomach and the body's *jatharagni* (the body's main store of fire for transformation, heating the body and penetration into crevices of the micro-body), diluting the acids that have been lying latent overnight in the stomach and pushing them onward and out, making room for and stimulating fresh hydrochloric acid and digestive enzymes that will be needed when a fresh load of food arrives. These slightly diluted acids also clean some of the sludge as they move forward through the intestines. This palmful of water is to be drunk before going to the bathroom and proceeding with the day.

As warm water provokes the flow of the intestines downward in a gentle peristalsis, it sometimes evokes a strong gastrocolic reflex, wherein stimulating the stomach reflexively stimulates the lower colon such that the bowels want to be emptied. When done between 3 and 7 a.m., during the *vāta* hours, it can augment and correct the flows of healthy *vāta*. Try it and see if it works for you.

- Bend to touch the floor with your hands before getting out of bed.
- Drink a palmful of lukewarm or room-temperature water from your right hand upon rising. It should be boiled and stored overnight in a clean, shiny copper container.

~ • 3 • ~

Morning Ablutions

Upon his return from Cambridge to Calcutta (now Kolkata), my father decided to renovate a new house. We moved into the third floor apartment in Santoshpur, complete with a dingy small bathroom housing an Asian toilet. He had decided to install European toilets in all the bathrooms upstairs, and so we waited for extra renovations. That year, I suddenly insisted on attending school, since I desperately needed to accompany my sister. It was decided that if I were to go, I had to prepare—at the ripe age of three—to stop using diapers.

Among my early memories is my favourite aunt trying to teach me how to squat over the Asian toilet. It was a white porcelain oblong bowl with a rectangular border sunken into the ground, with a dark six-inch round hole at one end leading to the beyond. On the short sides of the oblong bowl were two nine-inch rectangular porcelain slabs with chequered cuts, on which adult feet could rest on dry land without slipping during the squat. Both the distance between the feet and the gaping hole were so big that I cried in fear. There could be no mistakes on this toilet. One slip and I could end up inside. Or worse, the precious toys in my pockets could fall out and then they would be gone. After several futile attempts, my aunt finally allowed me to squat nearby on a newspaper and then transported the droppings into the toilet and threw in copious amounts of water to flush them down.

In the village, we would sit atop a large earthen bowl—much like a large planter—with a large banana leaf inside, and then Maa would transport the bowl out to the pond. There was no wasting paper or using non-biodegradables, as the pond would simply spit them to the edge.

When the upstairs bathrooms in our city house were finished, my youngest aunt was eager to make me modern. She dreamed of going to America one day and thus arranged all things in her life to be able to do so. She decided to teach me how to sit on our new European toilets so that I would not fall in. It was a balancing act. I spent more time teetering back and forth, afraid of hitting the water, than I did preparing my bladder or bowels. The urge would disappear. My aunt was determined, as though this was an essential step for obtaining her passport. After a few days, whenever she would sit me on the toilet, I would get so frightened that the urge would go away. Eventually, she would take me off and the urge would re-emerge immediately. I would quickly grab a newspaper and squat on the floor, fully prepared that someone would inspect the excrement and flush it for me. Since I had done it this way since leaving diapers, it seemed more logical than wobbling for her atop a porcelain bowl. Finally, after many attempts and great determination on her part, I was able to use the sitting toilet and actually do what needed to be done. She was pleased. Eventually, my aunt moved to Nebraska.

The science of morning ablutions (ablution comes from the Latin roots *ab*: away, and *luere*: to wash or get rid of) is the most well-kept secret in the world. Even sexual practices feature in films, poetry and books, but bowel and urine habits remain clandestine acts that few media will feature. Even modern medical science, which revels in telling you how much coffee, chocolate, sex and alcohol you should consume, has not conducted studies to prove the correct ways to complete our morning purges. Āyurvedic wisdom, however, has a specific set of instructions.

From where do we learn our bathroom habits? When we are young children, a parent or caretaker removes our diaper or carries us to the place where we are supposed to empty our bladders and bowels. We watch them show us, we try to do the same, we teach our younger siblings, we revise and readapt when our organs grow mature and, hopefully, we spend some time getting to know the anatomy of the gates that open to release our waste.

udadamukho mutrasakrddhiksinābhimukhe nishi |
vācan niyamya prayatah samvītāngo vaguntitah ||*3*||
prabartayot prachalitam na tu yatnadudiryet |

After the natural urge to dispel urine and faeces arises of its own accord, a person should eliminate them, facing north if early morning and if still dark then facing south. Silently one should squat, covering the head with a cloth, attending to the urge commenced on its own and without initiating the urge by force.

Astānga Samgraha of Vāgbhata,
Sūtra-sthāna; chapter 3, sloka 3–4

Yoga practices specify that one should give in to natural urges in the morning, gazing north, sitting in a private place, not gazing towards auspicious objects and not sitting near cowsheds, altars, burial grounds, on trees, near fire or on naked ground. One should avoid places that are very dirty, in the centre of a road, heaps of mud or ash, places of assembly or cow dung heaps. One should tighten the abdominal muscles and do a brief *muladhara* contraction (of the pelvic floor muscles)

before release. To aid this, ancient urinals were designed to have men bend on one knee to urinate. The closer we are to squatting, the more easily we release fluids and solids from our bladder and bowels.

The complications of conducting a randomized, double-blinded and placebo-controlled clinical trial (RCT) on the vast potential benefits of squatting vs sitting as we empty our bowels are significant. The methodology would be difficult to blind and to find a placebo would be comical! Anything that could be proven, like most non-drug interventions, would be easily questioned for the true conclusion of the study. In fact, RCTs bias all science towards drugs that can be masked, not lifestyle interventions. But without an RCT, how is any medical conclusion credible or reputable? Without from the funding National Institute of Health does anyone who is trained in science believe the research?

Nonetheless, clinicians without scientist credentials and titles have continued to propose that squatting aids the positioning needed by the pelvis for the best evacuation. The physiology of the nerves and the muscles of the bladder and bowels are most easily aided by the natural curve created by squatting and separating the thighs maximally. The muscles holding the rectum closed become relaxed upon squatting, and elimination is more complete. Haemorrhoids that occur from straining are relieved with squatting. The lower limbs receive regular exercise and have better tone and more flexibility. Varicose veins are minimized. There is no contact of the buttocks or thighs to a seat that could be unhygienic. Squatting also seals the ileocecal valve, located between the colon and small intestine, and allows the functions of the two areas to remain distinct. It avoids pressure on the uterus when using the toilet and may even reduce the occurrence or severity of diverticulosis. Since the logic of physiology does not count as evidence-based medicine, no one in the conventional world pays attention to it.

In the 1925 text, *The Culture of the Abdomen*, author Frederick Hornibrook states that medical authorities of the time were outspoken about the flawed new sitting toilet designed just decades earlier by cabinet-maker Joseph Bramah and plumber Thomas Crapper. Sitting toilets emerged in Europe where there was no orderly disposal of human waste, as there had been for millennia in Japan, India, Iran and countries with ancient civilized cultures. They commented on the toilet's faulty design and suspected health consequences, including constipation, hernias, varicose veins, haemorrhoids and appendicitis. A footstool was invented to alleviate the pressure on the pelvic muscles by elevating the feet. But the sitting toilet was convenient for the dresses of Europe, with their pockets and tight fittings. Also, the chair toilet spoke to the European love of monarchy; Henry VIII had a sitting toilet constructed for him after he had become obese. But with the wars at the turn of the twentieth century, replacing the chair toilet was a low priority and often financially not viable. A generation was created that preferred the chair, not learning how to manage their clothes during squatting.

In the US and western Europe, manufacturers quickly adapted to this preference, as it required more porcelain, several parts to assemble and thus rendered more profit. Companies in America no longer offer squatting toilets, and homes with Asian toilets are valued lower.

In the past decade, however, interest in health has redirected attention to squatting vs sitting while emptying the bowels. There are now companies that make platforms that fit around the sides of sitting toilets to create an elevated platform to squat. But, in the West, the sitting toilet persists.

- Squat to evacuate your bowels, especially if you have constipation or difficulties clearing your bowels.

Medical school does not explain why some people wake up and empty their bowels within the first half hour of sitting up, yet others go a few times a week. 'Normal variation' is the answer given by professors to cleanly tuck away the questions of naïve yet perceptive medical students whose questions linger. Āyurveda has observed patients for thousands of years, using clinical experience with humans, not mice and rats, as its foundation for evidence-based conclusions. Āyurveda argues that science is based on keen observations and clear perceptions, not blind dogma.

Āyurveda asserts that the *dosha*s that predominate in a body determine, the quantity, quality and frequency of a person's bowel movements. A *vāta* person, whose body qualities resemble the mobility and dryness of air and ether, has frequent, light and irregular bowel movements. Often, they have constipation. In later life, incontinence of bladder and bowel can occur. A *pitta* person, whose qualities resemble the goal-oriented and quick digestion of the transformation-themed elements of fire and water, has clean, quick, regular movements each morning just after waking. A *kapha* person—whose qualities resemble the heavy, slow and oily nature of water and earth—has slow, stodgy and infrequent bowel movements. However, most people do not have singular *dosha* body types. Over 80 per cent of people have two *dosha*s that predominate, such as *kapha–pitta* or *pitta–vāta*. Hence, schedules often vary from the above descriptions.

A *pitta–vāta* person will generally have clean, regular movements each morning, but witness fluctuations when *vāta* is elevated due to emotions, overwork or anger. This is because of the primary *pitta* nature, followed by the irregularity of the secondary *vāta* nature. A *vāta–pitta* person will generally have constipation and-or frequent movements of an irritable bowel that feel dry and incomplete or hot, especially when the person is unbalanced, has not eaten optimally the previous day or is angry. This is due to the airy nature that dries the colon and the mind and makes the body prone to *vāta* imbalances because of the combination of the heat of *pitta* and wind of *vāta*.

Like this, every combination of *dosha*s in a person predicts a type of bowel movement, recorded when sages wrote the classical texts. These apply even today, when Āyurvedic physicians accurately interrogate their patients. The correlation is uncanny and highly unlikely to be random.

If you have sluggish bowel movements and are storing waste in your bowels—which is thought to promote toxin and residue accumulation, abnormal bowel flora and gas—drink a mug of freshly boiled very warm water every morning just after awakening, before you eat or drink anything else. For the second serving, you may add fresh ginger to increase the digestive fire gently, but only if you are not prone to acid reflux. This warm water will clean your mouth and osophagus, and stimulate your gastrocolic reflex, urging flow down and out.

Āyurveda advises that it is best to rid the body of waste as soon as possible in the morning. Proper elimination from the colon and bladder ensures your body's proper functioning. If you wait until later in the morning or the day, you are slowly poisoning yourself due to accumulation of lingering toxins and waste, and creating an opportunity for chronic conditions to arise.

- If you have sluggish bowel movements, drink a mug of freshly boiled, very warm water every morning as soon as you awaken, before you eat or drink anything else. Add fresh ginger to the second serving, but only if you are not prone to acid reflux.
- Rid the body of waste as soon as possible in the morning.

Like sexual practices, no one wants to discuss the specifics of bowel habits, but everyone wants to know. Having a father who was a spermatologist, I have become well versed in finding words that explain intimate concepts without being too intrusive. Asking patients about their bowels has become a casual matter that requires tenderness to bring out needed information. Since medical school in the 1990s was highly inadequate in training us to take the sexual or bowel evacuation history of a patient, I found myself defaulting to the conversations I had overhead in my father's offices. Over the years, these questions have translated into a format in the patient intake form that I use to stir up the patient's awareness and learn about his/her body's daily news on the previous day's digestion activities.

In and Out: How You Process Food

Frequency of your bowel movements: Once a day/Several times a day/Once every ____

Regularity: Regular/Irregular

Colour: White/Yellow/Mid-brown/Has blood/Dark brown/Black/ Other ____________

Shape: Long like a banana/Like a pencil/In pieces/Has stringy pieces/Like pellets/Other ________

Density: Floats/Floats then sinks/Sinks/Formed like oatmeal/ Other __________________

In medical school, we learnt to ask about bowel movements in a very cursory manner. 'How are your toilet habits?' 'Fine . . . normal', the patient usually replied. That was it. A checkbox was marked on the patient's chart, and things moved forward. Since most people are not aware of a variety of toilet habits, how do we know what is normal? Only after extensive dialogue with a gastroenterologist was I able to learn that 'normal' is an impotent answer to questions about bowel function. Our intestinal wastes are one of the most potent sources of feedback our body gives us, but conventional medicine often ignores its importance.

Āyurveda uses very detailed interpretation and advice about bowel movements and waste. Called *purisha pariksha*, the observation of stool is one of ten examinations of the body in the art of Āyurvedic physical diagnosis. Likewise, *mutra pariksha* is observation of the urine and interpretation of the body based on its colour, thickness, presence of bubbles, smell and ability to attract ants. *Purisha* can be translated as 'that which occupies the lower channel of flow in the body', called the *pakwashaya*. It serves the purpose of keeping the intestines from collapsing, providing moisture and preserving heat, and thus should not be treated as only accumulated toxins and wastes. *Purisha* should be a shade of brown, come out in one long piece similar to the shape of a banana and be formed and intact. In water, it should float or hover in the upper portion of the toilet water. A spontaneous need to evacuate in the early morning is considered a good sign of *agni*, the body's healthy digestive fires. The lower belly should feel light when one is finished. Repeat visits should not be needed. Variations from this are interpreted clearly by Āyurveda, indicative of imbalanced *vāta, pitta, kapha, āma* (undigested material, residue and toxins stuck in the body) or *agni*.

❧

~•4•~

Washing Hands

After waking and thinking about my belly, I go into autopilot mode, having learnt early-morning chores from my mother since soon after infancy. I listen to my belly, touch the ground, get out of bed and head to the bathroom to complete morning ablutions, and then conduct a quick routine cleansing of the sensory organs.

Before the cleansing begins though, I wash my hands vigorously, not only because it is after I have gone to the toilet, but because it is the organ that will cleanse the others. On a morning in my lazy tween years in Omaha, I had awoken and chatted with my mother as we wandered to the bathroom together, engrossed in conversation. Without thinking, I had cupped my hands, filling them with water to wash my face, when she halted me with an admonition. 'You must first wash your hands, before even venturing to touch your face!' Immediately, in true adolescent spirit, I had challenged her to explain why. She had quoted the Gita, telling the tale of the five senses, masked as the five Pandavas. These strong warriors protecting our body must be cleaned and nurtured. Washing the hands ensures that the senses do not receive the dust and dirt of the hand's travels across life, sleep and the adventures of a curious child.

❧

snātah kshudvān viviktastho dhautapādakarānanah | 36

Food is to be ingested only after bathing and washing the hands, legs and face.

Astānga Hrdaya of Vāgbhata,
Sūtra-sthāna; chapter 8, sloka 36

❧

In ancient times, Āyurveda was aware of the importance of the concept of hygiene. Because it was recommended to empty bowels and bladder in nature, then cover it with earth in a secluded space, there was often no water body nearby. This necessitated conscious attention to obtaining water. A person would be seen leaving the house in the morning with a litre vessel of water in hand and a cloth over the shoulder. This indicated she/he was going towards a secluded area for the morning ablution rituals. Upon finishing cleaning the anal area, some water would remain for washing first the left, soiled hand and then for washing the other hand. Perhaps the term soiled derives from the practice of using a bit of mud to clean the anal area first with the left hand before washing it with water.

The hygiene of hand washing is related to the practice of drinking water by making a cup from the folded fingers and the palm of the right hand. The personalized measure of this volume is called a half *anjali*. Hand washing thus became a frequent precursor of anything that involved measuring, drinking or using the hands for the intake of any substance.

❧

prakshālanam hi pānyoshcha padayoh śuddhikāranam |
malashrama haram vrshyam cakshushyam rāksasāpaham||

The hands, mouth and feet should be thoroughly washed with soap and water after defecation.

Yoga Ratnakara of Mayūrapāda Bhiksu;
circa 1700 CE

Rāksa-ghna refers to microbes and antiseptic powers. Hands that are not properly washed allow microscopic eggs that can withstand water and a little soap to enter the gut and cause worm infestation. Hands and feet should be washed after removing waste from the eyes, ears and nose; after cutting hair; before and after eating food; after rising from bed; before performing worship activities; and after coming home from outside. In the absence of a bathroom, a person should squat or sit and wash the hands and feet on open ground while looking towards the east or north.

- Hands and feet should also be washed after removing waste from the eyes, ears and nose; after cutting hair; before and after eating food; after rising from bed; before worship; and after coming home from outside.

A large advance in public health and hygiene occurred in the western world when they recognized the importance of hand washing in the early 1900s. Prior to that, doctors and nurses in western hospitals would travel from patient to patient without cleaning their hands. The discovery transformed the practices that were developing to shape modern medicine, modern surgery, and their ideas of germ theory and cell theory supported hand washing to rid germs.

People in the West move from the streets to the dining table, without washing hands, much less cleaning the face, feet and mouth. The same shoes that track in dirt from the street are worn at the dining table. Hygienic practices now include hand sanitizer alcohol bottles and paper napkins, both of which are not good for our ecosystems of the earth and of the body. But they prevent some bacteria from entering the body, substituting them with preservatives and synthetic chemicals that are life-effacing.

Āyurveda considered these issues millennia earlier, developing copper bowls for storing water, saving clean rain water, boiling water from water bodies such as ponds and lakes and using water to clean the body more than any other substances. The concept of rinsing with water before and after taking anything into the personal sphere of the body became a daily practice and a filter of protection.

Today, while water is plentiful, diseases are on the rise due to lack of conscious hygiene and lack of technology to support clean water habits and ecosystems. From the rivers, to the sewage systems, to the toilets, to the personal use of water, an overhaul in your thinking about water usage will slowly shift you back to luscious, healthy living that will neither pollute the waters and dry your body, nor allow unnecessary infections. When you come in contact with clean water, you return to that wisdom, charging yourself with the energy of real clean, without the paper, detergents and chemicals promoted by the modern world.

❧

~ • 5 • ~

Washing the Face and its Orifices

Since a very young age, I watched my mother, aunts and elders wash their faces in the morning with clean, cold water. No soap, scrubs, brushes, washcloths or other tools; just a series of rinses. That is how I began. During the adolescent years, I was introduced to unperfumed clean soap only for the oily spots and never the neck or eyes. Oily dirt was removed only with oil, ghee or water. A few years later, I rediscovered sandalwood soap for summer and olive oil soap for winter. These soap bars were kept away from hand washing during the day and not used for bathing. Liquid soap had extra chemicals, including sodium lauryl sulfate for foaming, so I avoided it. If something traumatic like a pimple happened, we immediately rushed to the kitchen and applied turmeric, lemon or yogurt for 5 minutes and then applied fresh sandalwood paste at night. If the skin turned red from sun, heat, trauma, a scratch or tired late nights, cucumber or the cold cream from fresh raw milk would be applied; then ghee at night for nourishment and inner cooling.

Condition	Remedy
Pimple	Turmeric/lemon/yogurt, followed by sandalwood paste at night
Redness from heat, trauma or tiredness	Cucumber slice or paste and, cold cream from fresh raw milk, followed by ghee at night

Just after washing our hands, Āyurveda describes the specific processes by which we should clean the five sensory receptors early in the morning before we start our day of interacting with the five subtle energies—called *tanmatra*s—so that we can perceive them optimally and accurately.

Soon after awakening, first splash the face with cold water. Āyurveda does not recommend soap or other cleansers first thing in the morning unless there is excessive sweat or oil from heat or dirt that accumulated in the night. Cold water closes the pores for the day ahead, when dirt and grime can enter more easily. This may seem like an obvious task to some, but many people do not rinse their faces with water when they awaken, rather opting to do it during the shower.

After putting water on the face, work downward through the openings. The eyes should be rinsed first, many times with cold water. Some water should then be gently snuffed into the nose and immediately expelled. Swish some clean water in the mouth and throw it out.

- On awakening, splash the face with cold water. Avoid soap or other cleansers first thing in the morning, unless there is excessive sweat or oil from heat or dirt that accumulated in the night.
- After the face, rinse the eyes many times with cold water.
- Then gently snuff some water into the nose and immediately expel it.
- Swish some clean water in the mouth and throw it out.

Many modern consumers are convinced by the media that many products for the face are better than less intervention. If companies would explain the chemistry of their products more objectively rather than cloak it under trade-secret claims, people could make more intelligent decisions. Āyurveda's simple logic, unencumbered by marketing dollars to propagate its messages, looks at the biology and chemistry of the face.

There are a host of natural bacteria that live all over the healthy human body, known as the microbiome. On the skin, a subset of these 900 trillion bacteria, which balance our 100 trillion human cells, take up space so that harmful bacteria cannot invade. By overusing antibacterial creams, the skin loses its capability to produce its natural antibiotics that communicate signals and protect us. Alcohols and astringents in face care products dry the protective layer and kill the bacteria but make it easier for harmful bacteria to move into the cracks. When the skin is exposed to these artificial creams, it loses its tone and firm connection with the underlying live skin cells, fat, nerves, muscles and connective tissue called fascia—promoting wrinkles. Āyurveda classifies all astringents as chemicals made of the master elements earth and air, which are ultimately drying and increase *vāta*. When people dry their skin regularly, they create permanent *vāta* imbalances that can last a lifetime. The only temporary cosmetic solution is to apply moisturizers. This is very convenient for the facial products industry.

Modern science has confirmed in the past two decades that we absorb chemicals through our skin. Medicines that use this approach are called transdermal products. Painkillers and sedatives, nitroglycerin, contraceptive hormones and nicotine patches all send their chemicals directly into the bloodstream, which then circulate throughout the body to counter the effects that patients experience. Āyurveda also states that chemicals can be absorbed through the skin. Herbs and oils are delivered this way using medicinal protocols such as *panchakarma* (detoxification), *lepas* (herbal pastes) and *basti* (local oil pools made atop the skin). Therefore, all synthetic chemicals that have oily components, such as the petroleum derivatives in face washes and moisturizers, also get absorbed by the skin and eventually enter the bloodstream. Think about this—if you do not want to eat it, why would you put it on your skin? Companies that have their own sales in mind do not really care about your gut or skin. As long as the animals did not die in the preclinical lab studies that the Food and Drug Administration (FDA) requires, they are happy.

Āyurveda recommends that you gently rub or pat your face dry with a natural fibre cloth after washing it with cold water. Over weeks, your face will naturally become less greasy overnight, as it stops overcompensating in anticipation of the morning's alcohol, soap or astringent treatments.

If you feel very uncomfortable with the oily layer or it is grimy, use the following ingredients to cleanse. Āyurvedic beauty spas use them in a host of routines for the face.

Substance	Benefit	Application
Ghritkumari (Aloe vera)	It regenerates and soothes the epithelial (top skin) layer. Aloe vera contains a naturally produced antibacterial and antifungal chemical.	Apply aloe vera juice to acne scars and drink some too
Sandalwood (white, not red)	It naturally evens out pores and bleaches blemishes. This leaves a light residue and a fragrance.	Grind the wood stick for 40 seconds on a wet grinding stone used only for the sandalwood. Apply the paste to the face each night before bed, putting more atop pimples and oily areas. Use it weekly in the summer because it tightens the skin naturally. Apply daily if you are an adolescent or eat a lot of meat.
Lemon	Lemon juice is an acid and an astringent that is great to spot onto acne.	Equal parts of lemon juice and rose water make a nice facial mask. A pinch of turmeric can also be added.

Substance	Benefit	Application
Rose water	It is very cooling and is great for inflammation on the skin. It is used to treat many types of dermatitis and is excellent for rosacea. But Āyurveda emphasizes that the underlying cause of inflammation in the gut must also be addressed for long-term results.	Apply directly to inflamed areas with cotton.
Cucumber	Cucumber has cooling properties. It is great for reducing swelling and puffiness, especially under the eyes.	Thin cucumber slices can be placed for 10–15 minutes on the eyes. Otherwise, a puree of cucumber can be used as a scrub. Leave your cucumber scrub from your favourite facial product line in a covered glass for 3 hours. If it does not look brown and squishy after this time of oxidizing, it probably contains preservatives.

Substance	Benefit	Application
Dhania (leaves of the coriander plant)	These leaves have a cooling effect.	The seeds are often ground and used in cooking, or soaked overnight in water and drunk the following morning to relieve excess *agni*. The leaves are grated and pressed, and the juice is applied to pimples that are red and swollen.
Yoghurt	This is an effective cooling agent. It has some properties of milk, but really more properties of the alcohol and fire produced by the fermentation of the bacteria lactobacillus. These alcohols are mildly alkaline and cause a reflex of acidification of the skin.	Yoghurt is generally mixed with cucumber or rose water and left on for only 10–15 minutes. It has a skin-tightening and moisturizing effect.

Substance	Benefit	Application
Ghee (when made properly, is clarified butter, derived four stages after pure milk has been harvested)	Pure, well-made ghee, from the milk of a healthy cow, is an effective moisturizer and common carrier of many Āyurvedic medicines. Only a few companies make proper ghee, not just organic but according to the ancient recipe for ghee.	Rub the eyelids and eyelashes with ghee to rejuvenate the eyes and cool them (only if there is no lurking infection).
Eranda (castor oil)	Castor oil makes eyebrows and eyelashes grow thicker. It is commonly also used as a laxative once a week. The oil is also combined with other digestive herbs into a formulation designed for *vāta anulomana* (sending unharmonious *vāta* down and out).	Apply it to the eyebrows and near eyelashes at night. In the morning, remove it with some yogurt and lemon rind. As a laxative, ingest a teaspoon before sleep.

Replacing your bathroom cabinet contents with oils, spices, a mortar and pestle, and some small stone bowls will change your facial skin in a few months and be an investment for life.

Over several weeks of gradually diminishing use of artificial products, the skin's natural oils and incessant desire to rejuvenate come forth. Most people notice the natural, healthy glow.

~ • 6 • ~

Cleaning the Teeth

The bathroom cabinet was a chaotic place in all our houses, with many children, cousins, constant visitors, aunts and uncles, and regular travelling. My mother tried cups, shelves and sink-side vessels shaped like frogs, sea animals and various mermaids to make it pretty, to distinguish the different items and minimize hygiene errors. With five or more people using the bathroom for 2–3 brushing episodes daily, it was a challenge to discern whose items were whose.

As children, we did not own much in the house we called our own; music, books, rooms, beds, coats, cups, blankets, towels and plates belonged to everyone. In fact, many Indian languages do not have a verb for ownership or belonging, and it is translated as *mere paas hain*. 'It is near me'. But a toothbrush was one of the few things that was individual, and no one else used it or had the right to touch or move it.

Once, when we were travelling to our village, I had forgotten my toothbrush. I feared the implications of not being able to report the completion of morning chores, which incurred large penalties at home. Maa led me—not perplexed—outside to a dark, elegant tree with serrated leaves. She reached up and broke off a thin branch, removed the leaves and split the branch along its length into two. She then bit the end of the branch and flattened it as it splayed out like bristles attached to the dark wood. She showed me how to do the same, and then we inserted our bristled neem branch along our gum line and against our teeth, always brushing our lower row of teeth first. It was unforgettably bitter and left no minty aftertaste. She brought a cup of water and leaning my mouth upward, poured a bit in, careful not to touch the rim to my mouth. I swished a few times and spat out the old night with each mouthful. Then we sipped some hot water, and morning brushing was done.

Years later, we travelled to our farm in rural Nebraska and were trapped in a snowstorm. Again, we had no toothbrushes. I felt the discomfort of a grungy mouth. Maa came in smiling and poured into our palms some baking soda and a mixture of ground cinnamon, cardamom and clove powder that she kept in that house. We wet our pointer finger and used the powder mixture as a gritty tooth and gum cleaner. It worked well enough and satisfied my mother's requirements. We swished around and then sipped some fresh hot water.

It made we wonder why we were taught that sweetened, fluoride, menthol-laden toothpaste is considered the standard and superior way of cleaning teeth. In fact, it was only when Unilever and Colgate introduced their toothpastes through the power of television advertising that we were introduced to sweetness in toothpastes as a norm. The American Dentistry Association did not question the sugar and focused instead on the fluoride debate, which was alive in the 1940s. They quietly also mention on their website that toothpaste is one of several types of 'dentrifice', which includes pastes, gels and rarely seen powders.

❧

In Babi's veterinary collection are many books on animal preventive care. Every book spent a chapter on the care of the animal's mouth, none of which advocated brushing their teeth. They do not need dentures in the later part of life and nor do their teeth fall out.

It made me ponder that the elderly in India, and animals, usually keep their teeth until death. Was it the refined sugar in the diet—a new invention of the modern world in too much of a hurry for plant sugar to dissolve—that created cavities, or the sweeteners in the toothpaste, the fluoride, or some combination of modern uses that was not prevalent in Āyurvedic advice?

The promotion of fluoride in toothpastes began in the 1950s, as a novel idea for using the toxic surplus found in the slag that accumulated near mines where halogens were a byproduct of aluminum and metal ore refinement.

It was found that fluoride may have a beneficial effect on teeth, since it binds calcium, and the US government precipitously approved widespread public health measures to encourage mass consumption of it. This conveniently allowed the companies that had previously struggled to dispose of their waste to now sell it as a wanted marketable ingredient of chemical companies specializing in toiletries and household products.

To keep the chalky grit palatable, sugar and emulsifiers were added to keep it somewhat smooth and flowing in the tube. Pastes, gels and ointments were tried. Focus groups revealed that people equated foam with cleanliness, so sodium dodecyl sulfate (SDS) was added, exempted from any ban by the 1938 Food, Drug and Cosmetic Act in the US. Since a majority of Indian health and drug laws were copied verbatim from British health laws in 1940 and 1945, with blind adoption of US drug development laws over the past twenty years, SDS has made its way into most toothpastes in India, including Āyurvedic toothpastes. However, the Lifestyles of Health and Sustainability (LOHAS) demographic of highly educated, affluent and health-conscious consumers have demanded SDS-free, non-toxic options, which are now increasingly available.

Modern toothpastes have the following components: abrasives, fluoride, humectant, thickening binder, flavouring, preservatives and foaming detergent. Mild abrasives serve to remove debris in a majority of tooth powders. Some also remove residual surface stains. Today's toothpastes use calcium carbonate, magnesium carbonate, calcium phosphate dihydrate, chalk, alumina, dehydrated silica gels, hydrated aluminum oxides, phosphate salts and silicates. Āyurveda uses a coarse ground spice, such as cinnamon or clove, and/or micro-abrasion of natural bark appropriate to the season.

Fluoride is used with the claim that it strengthens tooth enamel and re-mineralizes tooth decay. All toothpastes approved by the American Dental Association (ADA) do contain fluoride. The fluoride debate rages in waves, since the American public ignores evidence available at the Environment Protection Agency (EPA) and websites that promote transparency. One of them cites a JAMA article, from 18 September 1943, which states that fluorides are general protoplasmic poisons. They inhibit enzyme systems, and water containing 1 ppm or more fluoride is undesirable. This was the AMA's stand on fluoridation until the US Public Health Service (PHS) endorsed nationwide fluoridation of the water, shortly after a lawyer of one of the largest producers of hazardous fluoride waste was appointed as the head of the US PHS in 1947. Many claim that the results of studies done under his leadership are skewed and were conducted without informed consent.

Few toothpastes are available today containing no sweetener, fluoride or SDS. The chemicals used to fluoridate 90 per cent of public drinking water are industrial-grade hazardous wastes captured in the air pollution control scrubber systems of the phosphate fertilizer industry, called silico-fluorides. Āyurveda never saw a benefit in diverting chemical wastes into people's mouth cleaners and instead chose to use spices and herbs.

The third component of modern toothpastes is some type of humectant to prevent water loss, such as glycerol, propylene glycol or sorbitol. The fourth component is a thickening agent or binder to stabilize the toothpaste. These include mineral colloids, natural gums, seaweed colloids and synthetic cellulose. Āyurveda used twigs and powders. Tooth powders do not require water, thickeners or binders and last for decades, much past the government-issued expiry stamp date, and fresh sticks do not require stabilization or artificial humectants.

The fifth component is a flavouring agent, such as saccharin or other non-natural sugar sweetener to provide taste. Dentists choose to quietly ignore the contradiction between this and their simultaneous campaign to stop eating sweets and sugary candies that cause cavities. On paper, flavouring agents must not promote tooth decay. Āyurveda recommends the benefits of bitters and astringents in mouth cleaning as these chemicals generally are naturally antibacterial and antifungal, and dry the mouth and reduce *kapha*. Experiencing all six tastes in the day also properly stimulates all components of the salivary glands. Colouring and preservatives are added to preserve shelf life.

The last component of modern toothpastes is detergent to create foaming action and include sodium lauryl sulfate, also known as sodium dodecyl sulfate, or sodium N-lauryl sarcosinate. These chemicals have been banned in many countries, as a result of incriminating evidence and safety data.

There are two kinds of people in the world: those who use tooth powder, and those who use toothpaste. At different times of the year for different climates, Āyurveda specifically advocates the use of different powders, made of coarse ground spices that are part of our diet and will not poison us if swallowed. If twigs are out of season or unavailable, Āyurveda recommends powders of ginger, black pepper and long pepper, known as *trikatu*; or the powder of three powerful fruits that are commonly used to detoxify the blood and liver, known as *triphala*. These powders are ideally applied with the finger, so we can feel the crevices and ridges inside the mouth, increasing body awareness.

Āyurveda recommends a panoply of spices for cleaning the mouth. The plants and twigs of woods should be either *kashaya* (astringent), *katu* (acrid/pungent), or *tikta* (bitter). Common ones include *darchini* (cinnamon), neem (*Azadirachta indica*), *babul* (*Acacia nilotica*), *arka* (*Calotropis gigantea*), *khadira* (*Acacia catechu*), *karañja* (*Pongamia pinnata*), *kakubha* (*Terminalia arjuna*), *madhuka* (*Madhuca longifolia*) and *nyagrodha* (*Ficus bengalensis*).

Use is based on the season, *dosha, rasa* and *virya* of the day. Experiencing taste is important, as it changes the composition of the saliva. Cinnamon can be used all throughout the year, as it is a sweet astringent that is favourable for the spring and summer, and its pungent heating qualities are favourable for autumn and winter. More sour and salty tastes are recommended for spring. Neem is the best of the bitters and is excellent for the late winter and spring seasons as it cuts *kapha* and lowers *pitta*. *Khadira* is advised for the *kapha* cold season, as it is an astringent, which dries the oily nature of *kapha* and also decreases *kapha* and *pitta* as it is composed of the cooling and drying elements of earth and air. *Madhuka* is excellent for the hot, windy season because its sweet and emollient properties lower the heat, decreasing the *pitta* and *vāta* effects of the season. *Karañja* is the best among pungent plants and is used in the rainy season, when both the heat of *pitta* and dampness of *kapha* are high.

For centuries of decades, Āyurveda has advised people on how to care for their teeth if they do not have time or access to powders, with the use of fresh twigs being the most traditional. The instructions are very specific; after eating at night and early in the morning, use fresh twigs devoid of branches and knots, grown in rich soil; pick a new twig every day; find twigs as thick as a little finger and approximately twelve centimetres or five inches long; brush from bottom to top, as deposits tend to flow downward; rinse the mouth with clean water from a fresh river or water that was boiled the night before and kept in a copper vessel to cool overnight.

Some old-style toothpaste companies in the West continue to promote pure baking soda, used widely before industrialization. In India, Āyurvedic spices are commonly marketed as the cornerstone for medicinal dental preventive care, adding 'modern' components to compete with mainstream toothpastes. While tooth powder remains available in most Indian groceries, the convenience, charm and advertising placement of toothpaste has won.

To take best care of the teeth:

- After eating at night and early in the morning, use fresh twigs of neem or babul.
- Pick a fresh new twig every day, as thick as a little finger and approximately twelve centimetres or five inches long.
- Brush from bottom to top, as deposits tend to flow downward.
- If there is existing disease in the mouth has active disease, rinse it with clean water boiled the night before and kept in a clean shiny copper vessel to cool overnight.

Use the following herbs as tooth powders in their correct seasons:

- Cinnamon can be used all throughout the year, as it is a sweet astringent that is favourable for the spring and summer, and its pungent heating qualities are favourable for autumn and winter.

- More sour and salty tastes are recommended for spring.
- Neem is the best of the bitters and is excellent for the late winter and spring as it cuts *kapha* and lowers *pitta*.
- *Khadira* is advised for the *kapha* cold season.
- *Madhuka* is excellent for the hot, windy season.
- *Karañja* is the best among pungent plants and is used in the rainy season.

Āyurveda advises some people to refrain from using toothbrushes or hard twigs in the morning as part of their daily routine, recommending only soft powders and their finger to clean their mouth.

This includes those who are suffering from severe indigestion or diarrhoea, have been spontaneously vomiting, have shortness of breath or asthma, severe cough, fever, facial paralysis, severe thirst, or ulcerations or inflammation inside the mouth, such as canker sores or cold sores. Āyurveda also discourages people to use brushes if they have heart disease, eye diseases, head conditions or diseases, and ear diseases.

On the surface, this recommendation may seem random to a modern medical scientist. However, Āyurvedic reasoning correlates with biochemistry. Clearing away bacteria in the mouth alters the ecosystems of different bacteria colonies around the body trying to re-establish balance. Digestive enzymes in the mouth are affected by connections from the mouth's taste receptors to the gut and gut–brain axis that connect the gut's immune system to the brain's hormones.

- If you suffer from severe indigestion or diarrhoea, have been spontaneously vomiting, have shortness of breath or asthma, severe cough, fever, facial paralysis, severe thirst, or ulcerations or inflammation inside the mouth such as canker sores or cold sores, refrain from using toothbrushes or hard twigs, and use only soft powders and a finger to clean your mouth.
- Also avoid brushes if you have heart disease, eye diseases, head conditions or diseases, and ear diseases.

Physicians do not learn much about the teeth and gums during medical school. For a few days in anatomy and radiology, we do learn about the mandible as a fulcrum for balancing the cranium or skull atop the spine. It seems obvious that the balance of the jaw is a fundamental part of good balance, neck flexibility and functions of the nerves that flow through the canal of the head spine. The balance of the jaw in turn depends on the outermost place where it rests: the teeth, specifically the bite. It is therefore imperative that the teeth are anchored well and interlock properly.

The field of neuromuscular dentistry explores this relationship. Placement of the bones and the way they sit atop each other is also explored in other bodywork sciences, such as Feldenkrais, osteopathy and chiropractic. Āyurveda promotes proper placement of the gums and teeth via yoga postures that strengthen the neck, jaw and posture. In my dozens of annual visits to conventional dentists, I have never experienced one who looks at the alignment of my teeth and bite with my jaw, eyes and spine. Yet, good Āyurvedic doctors and holistic dentists observe the symmetry and work with this obvious relationship as part of head and neck health.

❧

My mother never taught me to floss. The dentist did. My mother taught us to rinse our mouths each and every time just after we ate. She would then give us a glass of water to drink about 20 minutes after our meal. When we entered the American school system, we would leave the cafeteria and go directly to a classroom. I asked my mother where I was supposed to rinse, and she told me to go to the bathroom every time after lunch and wash my mouth and hands, and urinate if needed.

So, I would pause after lunch to go to the bathroom and rinse my mouth, urinate and then wash my hands. One day, a girl in the bathroom told me I was dirty and rude for spitting into the sink and that I was not supposed to put the bathroom water in my mouth. I was confused. The 'to dos' of India were forbidden and 'not to dos' in America. The world turned upside down as I was taunted continuously and ostracized, and I stopped rinsing my mouth after lunch.

Within a few years, I was taken to the dentist and found to have cavities that needed filling, and we were advised to chew gum to clean our mouths after lunch. Decades later, I now feel appalled at the blatant sense of misdirection propagated by modern cultures. People in ancient cultures rinse their mouths before and after their meals; they do not floss, and they do not lose their teeth.

❧

~ • 7 • ~

Cleaning the Tongue

Unlike the girls' bathrooms in our homes, my father's bathroom was filled with shaving supplies, hair oils, potions, colognes and Father's Day presents that sat there lovingly, but unopened. He had a cup for his toothbrush and toothpaste, a sharp, steeply curved silver spoon and a long U-shaped old copper instrument. Of course, I was too scared to ask for years because it could be a boy's tool. But finally, curiosity forced me to inquire, and I learnt about tongue scrapers.

I had been taught to brush my teeth and gums, to rinse my mouth several times, to gargle and to swish, but I had never scraped my tongue until adolescence. My mother explained that only after we started eating adult foods and began menstruating did we need to clean our tongues. She explained that if we stayed healthy and ate clean food at home, our tongues would be clean. If we fell ill or when we started working outside the house where the threat of outside toxins increased, we would start to accumulate stuff between our taste buds.

In high school, where I struggled to understand science and truth versus the reality inside our house, which was a kind of departure from America without a passport, I began to ask school friends about toothbrushes, gingerly approaching the topic of scraping the tongue. Some told me they gagged if they touched their tongues when they brushed. Some would vomit immediately if their tongue and toothbrush touched, they confessed readily. The biology teacher suggested that brushing the tongue with the toothbrush would stimulate the taste buds. But no one advocated scraping the tongue, and no one could understand my lack of fear in scraping my tongue after watching my mother for years. So, like many rituals of being an Indian American, the issue of tongue scraping became a mandatory, yet clandestine, act of daily living.

In our attempts to hide our different habits from visitors to our home in Omaha, my mother first hid her copper tongue scraper permanently in her red and orange rose toiletry travel bag. On a visit to Japan, after forgetting her tongue scraper, she found a sharply oblong unique silver teaspoon which worked beautifully to scrape her tongue. It worked so well that she tipped the housekeeper and purchased the spoon. Since then, that spoon resides in her bathroom cup. Soon after, I was given a similar spoon as a decoy for use in the American world, where tongue scrapers are ridiculed. The spoon travels with me now, as my reminder of living with a silver spoon.

Called *jihva nirlekhana*, Āyurveda recommends scraping of the tongue (*jihva*), not brushing it. Brushing stimulates the buds but does not clean them. The old minuscule morsels of food lie trapped in the crevices between tongue buds, like dirt at the bottom of the carpet between the thick loops of wool, creating toxins, lack of taste, bad taste and malodour. Āyurveda tells us to scrape the tongue to reduce oedema and stiffness of tongue as well, then rinse the mouth again.

Scraping the tongue properly is like combing hair—pressing down too hard will cause bleeding and too softly will be ineffective. A proper tongue scraper scratches but does not pierce. In the US, soon after I began recommending copper tongue scrapers, patients informed me that stores had stopped selling them because dentists had proclaimed they were dangerous, cutting people's tongues! When I inquired, there was a fear that people would cut their tongues on the sharp edges of the U-shaped scraper. It seemed obvious that people needed to modulate how hard they pressed the scraper on the tongue, but grocers retreated, purchasing the newly created American plastic scrapers instead.

Āyurveda recommends the use of a silver or copper scraper, as silver lowers *pitta* and heat, and copper reduces the congestive build-up of *kapha* and counters the inflammation seen in *pitta*. Hence, these are the ideal metals for tongue scraping and other instruments for the head and face.

jihvā-nirlēkhanaṁ raupyaṁ sauvarṇaṁ vārkṣamēva cha |
tanmalāpaharaṁ śastaṁ mṛdu ślakṣṇaṁ daśāṅgulam ||13||
mukha-vairasya daurgandhya-śōphajāḍyaharaṁ sukham |
danta-dārḍhyakaraṁ rucyaṁ snēha-gaṇḍūṣha dhāraṇam ||14||

To scrape the tongue, use an instrument made of silver, gold, iron or the strong twig of a tree that is soft, smooth, ten fingers long and serves to clean. ||13||

This removes bad tastes and odour in the mouth, cures oedema, stiffness of the tongue and returns the sense of taste. Holding oil still in the mouth strengthens and whitens the teeth. ||14||

Suśruta Samhita,
Cikitsā-sthāna; chapter 24, sloka 13–14

- Use a tongue scraper rather than a brush to clean your taste buds and to reduce oedema and stiffness of the tongue.
- Use a silver or copper scraper rather than a plastic one.

❧

Modern medicine discovered the gustatory receptors for taste recently, which got more attention when the Nobel Prize was awarded to Professors Linda Buck and Richard Axel at Columbia University for their work on the mechanism of action of olfactory receptors for smell. Smell receptors overlap significantly with gustatory sensation, connecting air-bound chemicals from the food we are about to taste.

Modern science knows five tastants: sweet, sour, salty, bitter and umami. Umami is a Japanese term that means delicious and corresponds to the glutamate receptor. It is triggered by tomatoes, potatoes and glutamic acid, which is found in savoury and meaty foods. Science has not classified pungency and astringency as tastes. Āyurveda distinguishes between tastes that draw lots of saliva into the mouth—pungent—and tastes that draw saliva out of the mouth—astringent.

The oral cavity contains between 3,000 and 10,000 taste buds in most adults. These taste buds have also been found in the antrum or upper stomach, and upper oesophagus as well as other parts of the digestive system, such as the pancreas and liver, with the likely function of coordinating digestive enzymes and elegant communication about the tastes soon arriving from the mouth. Taste buds are also found in the brain, on the palate of the mouth, the tonsillar pillars, the epiglottis and respiratory system, on the testicles and testes, the urinary bladder and on the anus. The taste receptors in the testicles may modulate the amount of sugar provided to the sperm, as fructose is both a poison and vital substrate for sperm motility.

Āyurveda conceives taste differently from the way these are defined in modern science. Every morsel, whether it is food, medicine, mineral, plant or animal, is made of the five great elements. These elements combine in dyads to produce a taste.

madhura (sweet)	*prthvi* + *jal*	downward roots (*apana vayu*), grounding
amla (sour)	*prthvi* + *agni*	both heavy and light
lavana (salty)	*jal* + *agni*	hydrates, moves, lightens and softens
katu (pungent)	*agni* + *vayu*	upward (*udana vayu*) aromatics; kills pathogens
tikta (bitter)	*vayu* + *akāsh*	promotes tastes of other food
kashaya (astringent)	*vayu* + *prthvi*	is drying and great for curbing the appetite

Each of these tastes triggers different fires in the mind, the tongue and upper stomach, which digest these tastes and absorb them selectively in special zones of the gut, according to the body's needs. As these tastes are absorbed, they provide fuel for the tissues to develop their elemental components. Thus, tasting each morsel is important for the correct digestive enzyme to be activated. Fat tissue requires more grounding and little heat, so it absorbs mostly sweet-tasting substances. Bones likes movement and flow, since blood courses through them all day. Hence, bones have an affinity for light substances and selectively absorb bitter and pungent substances. While this way of thinking is completely foreign to biochemical thinkers, it correlates quite well clinically with what we see in patients. Through Āyurveda, one can also make amazingly precise and accurate predictions about diseases from these correlations of tastes with tissues.

❧

In medical school, we learnt that the coating on the tongue is just there, randomly in some and not others. We open the mouth to look for swelling in the uvula (the thing that hangs down from the back of our throat), then we observe the tonsils and gums, and remove the tongue depressor. However, Āyurveda imparts great importance to the tongue—as an indicator of the state of digestion. The following are a few time-tested observations.

State of Tongue	Indication/Condition
Scalloping around the edges	Unabsorbed nutrients in the gut
Cracks on the surface	Chronic *vāta* problems in the colon
Thick white coating	Heaviness; *kapha* in the colon
Thick cheesy coating	Undigested *kapha* in the upper gut, usually the stomach; commonly seen during food poisoning or severe indigestion
Brownish, watery or gel-like coating	*Vāta* dominating the gut
Yellow or yellow–white coating on the red perimeter of the tongue (scraped off with a tongue cleaner but may build up again)	Heat and excess *pitta* in the gut, usually the small intestine

Āyurveda says these guidelines should be checked with cross-questioning of the patient about food habits, symptoms and bowel movements in the past 2 days.

❧

~ • 8 • ~

Water in the Morning

In each oven of our houses lives a copper vessel. We have had copper, brass and earthen vessels around us our entire lives, except for the Omaha years, when my father's work at Creighton had us living American and enjoying the wonders of Tupperware. My mother regularly boils *kachha jal* (raw water) to cook out the chemicals and unwanted energies, and then pours it into the copper vessel. The big vessel that lives in the largest oven in Princeton basks in the heat of the pilot lamp, which stays on all day and throughout the year in modern stoves in America. It keeps the water at a warm 27–32°C and is nice to drink in winter. In the morning, my mother drinks a large glass of water as soon as she enters the kitchen after her early-morning rituals.

Over the years, as we have aged, we have learnt to stoke our fire and burn our toxins using the simple wisdom of boiling our water. Either we drink it freshly boiled and hot to begin the day or we drink a glassful that has come to room temperature when the weather is hot or our *pitta dosha* is aggravated. Either way, we feed our body only the water that has been cleaned and primed for its journey into the living cells that make our body.

❧

sprstvā dhatun-malān-ashru vasā-keśa nakhāh cyutān ||8||
snātvā bhoktumanā bhuktavā suptvā ksutvā surārchhane |
rathyām ākramya ca acamet upavishta udangmukhah ||9||

Ācamana (in Sanskrit*, chama* is to sip) should be done after contact with inauspicious things like tissues such as blood, muscle or fat; excreta; tears; muscle fat, hair or nails of animals (fallen or cast off). It should also be done after bathing, at the beginning of the first sense of hunger, at the end of meals, during *suptvā* (waking up), after *ksutvā* (sneezing), before commencing the worship of God, after a chariot ride (*rathyā*), after a long walk or journey, and after the usual daily ablutions.

prāngmukho vā viviktastho na bahirjānu nānya drk |
ajalpan anuttarāsangī svacchaih angushta mulagaih ||10||
nauddhrtaihi na anato na urdhvam nāgnipakvaihi napūtibhih |

Facing north or east, *ācamana* should be done daily, squatting or sitting in an erect posture, in solitude and with full concentration and without speaking. Both hands should be positioned inside and below the knees, looking nowhere else, without talking, wearing an upper garment or cloth over the shoulder. The water should be pure, and first used to wash both hands, face and feet, and then the right hand to ensure it is clean. It is then poured from the left into the right palm at the root of the thumb, which will be cupped placing the thumb at the base between the middle and pointer fingers. It should be sipped three times without making any sound and without spilling.

na phenabulbudaksāraihi na aika hastārpitaih jalaih ||11||
na ardrai eka pānih na ama dhya hastapādo na śabdavan |

The water should not be twice boiled, should not have any bad *puti* (smell), *phena* (froth) or *bulbuda* (bubbles), and it should not have *ksāra* (alkaline) in it. Sipping of water is prescribed after cleaning the excreta, after tears, after taking a bath, after eating, after sleeping, after sneezing, after worship and after travelling.

Astānga Samgraha of Vāgbhata,
Sūtra-sthāna; chapter 3, slokas 8–12

❧

Water is discussed at length in several chapters of the classic texts. In the *dinacharya* chapters, Āyurveda describes the importance of water when we first awaken and just after we have listened to our gut and assessed how it feels, advising us to do *ācamana,* drinking a palmful of water from a cup made with the right hand. This first daily water sends a signal to the gut that the body has awoken from its quieted state during the night. At the end, we touch the *marma* (vital points) near the eyes, ears, nose, outer lips, temples and clavicles. After we clean our face and orifices, and emerge clean on the outside to start the day, we should drink a larger amount of pure water to clean ourselves on the inside. This water may be boiled and drunk hot, warm or cold, depending on the season, climate and the person's constitution and state of *agni*.

While modern medicine emphasizes the importance of drinking lots of water daily, recommending two litres a day to healthy adults, Āyurveda recommends we drink only what we are called to drink, sipping not guzzling, and being more aware of the purity of the water and its colour, smell and taste. It details the diseases to which we predispose ourselves when we drink water beyond what our body asks for—thirst, lethargy, flatulence, being overweight, cough, reduction in digestive power, nausea, salivation, difficulty in breathing and increased nasal mucous, describing a gradual increase in *pitta*, *kapha* and *āma* . Drinking too much water causes much of it not to be digested, thus contributing to disharmony of the body. To know what your body needs, talk to it every day. Drink less of any other fluid for a few days, and your body will tell you how much water it needs. Rather than listening to a doctor who does not take care of his/her own body, invite yourself to take a sip of water and see what aligning with water does for you.

- After drinking a palmful of water on waking, touch the *marma* (vital points) near the eyes, ears, nose, outer lips, temples and clavicles.
- After you clean your face and orifices, drink a larger amount of pure water. It may be boiled and drunk hot, warm or cold, depending on the season, climate and the person's constitution and state of *agni*.
- Drink a small amount of clean water after excretion, tears, bathing, after eating, sleeping, sneezing, after worship and travelling.
- Note how much water is optimal for you. Drink only that much, rather than a non-individualized prescribed amount.

❧

~ • 9 • ~

Auspicious Objects

In a hallway of every house where we have lived is a small closet that is one of the fanciest spaces of the house; it is the altar room. It is where we sit to meditate, pray every day at each sunrise and sunset, shed our worries, our tears, our excess emotions and offer the best of ourselves as we begin our day. As a child, I always knew where to find my mother early in the morning. She would sit cross-legged, with a burning candle and incense stick. There was no interrupting her, though we invented emergencies to get her attention and permission to leave the house to play. We were not allowed to touch certain sections of the altar room and as we got older, we were initiated into new duties and meanings of different objects and different rituals were explained to us.

The construction of an altar really requires just six objects, though dozens grew to find a home in our *thakurer ghor*s (worship house) over the years—a candle or source of light, something sweet smelling (such as incense or flowers), some water, a place for offerings, a grounding spot called an asana and an auspicious object. My mother used beautifully drawn pictures that symbolize the facets of human potential: wisdom, abundance, healing, love, wealth and perseverance. These pictures were the pantheon of deities that filled Hindu mythology. My mother explained that they were invented so that we could meditate on these qualities within ourselves, focusing on the symbols that showed themselves to us in the pictures. We were encouraged to focus on any picture we were drawn to and carefully observe every detail we could, using it to draw us into that part of ourselves that reflected that detail. During our school years, she would show us Saraswati, the goddess of learning and wisdom, emphasizing her calm gaze, her wise beauty, her simple elegance and the ever-present book in her hand. Over the years, as gifts, statues and calendars came into our home, they were in turn cleaned and placed humbly into the altar room. All flowers touched the altar and were offered there before they settled into a vase in any living room.

pranamya devān vrddhāmscha mangalāshtaśatam śūbham |
śrnvan kāñchanavinya*stam sarpih paśyodanantaram* ||*23*||

Gods and elders should first be worshipped, then the 108 auspicious names of God should be repeated while the person looks at his/her own image in a golden vessel filled with ghee.

Astānga Samgraha of Vāgbhata,
Sūtra-sthāna; chapter 3, sloka 23

Over the years, waking up and taking time to look at an auspicious object has become a deeply reverent practice of connecting with the inner self, before starting a busy day. In these early hours of *vāta*, when the air is light, sitting for a few moments with objects we love can inspire us and orient our inner compass to our day. The daily planner of our heart can register its vote on what really needs to be done. Getting centred has more value than just being religious: it is an ode to the inner self.

Āyurveda says we should locate our altar room in the north-east corner of our house. If this is not possible, an upper floor, rooftop or closet in which we can face north or north-east is ideal. Sometimes, all that is possible is a small shelf on the north or north-east wall or corner of the room, on which sits a candle, a small photo of a beloved deceased relative or our favourite deity. What is most important is to have a place where we can stop, settle our mind and be present for a moment or two early in the day. Without this focus, we run around all day with our minds disconnected from our bodies. Who wants to be on a highway with a car whose driver does not know where she/he is going? Vision is a powerful tool for orienting the mind. Therefore, Āyurveda says we should look at our parents or elders, beloved priests, the sacred fire, the sun, gold, a cow, ghee or clean water early in the morning to invoke thoughts that are auspicious.

- Altars in the home are best located in the northeast corner of the house.
- If this is not possible, use a shelf in the northeast corner of a room or an upper floor, rooftop or closet where you can face north or north-east.
- Nurture this space and use it to centre yourself.

In the years since neuroscience has evolved, the neurobiology of hope has provided inspiration on how and why to keep our moods positive. The emotions that our mind produce when we see inspirational stimuli produce neurotransmitters that promote health, whereas chronic negativity and hopelessness caused by failure, bullying and violence will decrease the neurotransmitters serotonin and noradrenaline, and cause abnormal functioning of the limbic system, where our emotions seem to be processed. It also causes a malfunction of the connections between our hypothalamus, pituitary and adrenals, causing a strong overdrive and output of cortisol, which suppresses the immune system.

In biomedicine, several drugs have been created to artificially increase serotonin levels in people who are depressed and feeling hopeless. Rather than studying which thoughts decrease serotonin and working to decrease such thinking, a drug prevents serotonin from being destroyed, thus increasing its levels in the brain. Clinically, we see a variety of effects from these serotonin drugs. Moods are lifted, but sometimes erratic behaviour emerges, or patients feel that something is controlling their mind. They often do not feel comfortable in their own bodies or in interactions with other people, and report being uncomfortable watching other people's emotions.

Psychotherapy uses behavioural changes, ritual exercises such as journaling and weekly appointments, mental analysis, awareness-building skills and a variety of tools for the psyche and mind to become stronger, so that it can harness the depressed mind and body and lift it.

Modern scientists recently discovered a way to conceive the mind to distinguish it from the brain. They profoundly 'discovered' what yoga shastra has been teaching for thousands of years; the mind is a modifiable lens through which we can perceive, process and regulate the functions of our body and processes of life. Using this empowered viewpoint, scientists are now developing tools to make the mind stronger, using contemplation, relationships and emotional intelligence. They are finding that conditioned, cultivated behaviour create mental and emotional changes that alter neurotransmitters and over time, transform and reshape the pathways of our nerve impulses, changing the way we think, respond, react and feel.

Scientists are finding that spirituality has a profound effect on the prefrontal cortex, the part of the brain that determines a host of behaviour, known as executive functions, such as decision-making, interaction with society, problem solving, judgment, focus and abstract skills required for integrating inner goals with implementation of thoughts and actions. It is also essential for the expression of personality. Scientists like David Perlmutter, Andrew Newberg and Daniel Siegel have all approached the questions of how the mind works and how we can get it to work better. Work on the role of neural mechanisms associated with religious and spiritual experiences is slowly revealing that faith, meditation, word choices, thoughts of kindness and actions of compassion improve brain health and actually condition the architecture of the brain.

Āyurveda takes a different approach because it integrates a person into the universe. Beginning at the same point clinically, where a person is feeling hopeless or depressed, Āyurveda prescribes first putting them in nature and letting them spend time observing the universe, with all its lessons and ultimate balance and awesome, unapologetic power. In addition, interactions are encouraged with small children and loved ones who will not judge them. They are integrated into household tasks to feel needed, and conversation with the family is used to engage them in relationships and communication, and to enable them to engage with their inner selves. They spend time daily in the morning and evening *sandhya*, guided by family and friends, looking at and touching auspicious objects while imbibing their energy, at the time when the natural changes in *vāta* from the change of the sun can best be used to change the mind. These rituals help the mind change track and awaken clearly to what the soul is trying to convey in its mission to move the body to its purpose. Once we have something that we align with in our core—some project, work or dream to fulfil—we have a task or reason for putting a foot forward towards tomorrow. Hopelessness can only be countered by hope.

Āyurveda also supports these depressed situations with nutrition and herbs that alter the *dosha*s. Since health is the balance of *dosha*s and *dhatu*s work in harmony to eliminate wastes and transform, move and stabilize the body, it follows that there is something off balance about a depressed person in his *dosha*s, *dhatu*s or *mala*. Āyurveda sets out to fortify the mind by first decreasing aberrant movements and flows of *vāta*. *Brahmi, jatamansi* and *shankapushpi* are commonly combined for their *vāta*-balancing properties and given with any of several herbs that will counter imbalances of *guna*s. When a person's digestive fire is corrected and in balance, the body can digest good nutrition, stabilizing the *sadhaka pitta*, the energy of transformation associated with will force that gives us determination and perseverance in the roughest of times.

As *vāta* and *pitta* are stabilized, the mind's *guna*s, or qualities, must also be addressed. Known as the *mahaguna*s, they are *sattva*, *rajas* and *tāmas*, developed in the ancient Indian system of philosophy called Sankhya. The lethargic or *tāmasic guna* is a necessary energy for the mind, as it needs to periodically disengage and rest. In excess, however, it promotes laziness, lethargy and depression. *Rajas* or the dynamic *guna*, promotes activity, curiosity and a do-er mentality, but it also promotes arrogance, egotistical narcissism and bullying. *Sattva* is the quality of harmony, balance and oneness with the environment. For more than half of our day, we should live with the quality of *sattva* dominating in our mind. However, too much *sattva* will prevent us from keeping boundaries from others and may lead to violations of our space by people who have not developed mentally and emotionally to be *sattvic*. Activities that cleanse the body of the *tāmas*, such as exercise, team sports and hiking in nature, are encouraged to dilute negative energies by infusing positive energies into the body through all inlets: food, sound, conversations, visual objects, smells, the sun and the environment that penetrates through our skin. As a person takes in the environment, it may change his/her mental composition, as we know emotions can change neurotransmitters, which alter hormone levels and the immune system.

During her *sandhya* pūja every day, my mother's ode to the change of light is accompanied by *arati*, blessings of light from the heat of a candle or oil lamp. Called *arātrika* in Sanskrit, meaning something that removes *rātri* (darkness), it is a ritual of worship, a part of pūja, wherein light is offered to the deities. It is a symbolic gesture of lighting our insides or enlightening our inner selves.

The entire ritual requires a series of offerings into a fire or in the direction of worship, usually facing north or north-east. Eight objects are offered sequentially, using clockwise motions, as symbols of the five elements of which we are made—ether/space, air/wind, fire, water and earth. Firstly, incense or *agarbatti* is offered, representing the smell and solidity of earth. It is followed by sprinkling water, and then burning a light or candle to honour the fire in us. Thereafter, a peacock fan is used to convey the qualities of air, movement and wind, followed by movements with a cow, horse or yak tail to offer acknowledgment of subtle ether or space. In addition, offerings are made using a *jal-shankh*, or water-filled conch shell that opens to the left, to symbolize water and liquidity. Blowing of a *shankh* (conch shell) represents sound and the ethers. A *trishul* symbolizes the magnetic forces in the ethers. A plate of flowers sprinkled with sandalwood represents the earth and its ever-new nature. New cloth of cotton or silk corresponds to the weavings of earth and fruit reminds us of the bounty of earth.

Though *arati* differs for occasions and cultures, it is very precise about providing auspicious offerings that symbolize our inner selves, to our inner selves symbolized by the deities.

~ • 10 • ~

Sweetness for the Day

As they each finished their early morning chores, my mother and father would emerge from the bathroom and immediately head to the altar room, to do a peculiar series of tasks. Though they seemed random, they were symbolic gestures that preceded anything that might invade their day. With swift and purposeful but automated steps, my mother would step from the altar room, look at the photos of her parents, long deceased during her young adolescence, whisper some words to them, smell a flower or some incense, recite a mantra and put a sweet raisin or grain of rice on her tongue. Then she would rush to begin her day.

My father would emerge freshly showered, enter the altar room and then emerge magically from his bedroom with fresh cologne, singing a mantra under his breath. He would look at photos of Rabindranath Tagore, Albert Einstein and Vivekananda, and then put a herb on his tongue or some drops of the water washing from the *Narayan shila*, called *charana-amrta*, or washings from the feet of the Lord.

Decades later, now after his stroke, he still emerges from his room, pauses at the altar, as he sniffs the incense strongly, and his lips move slightly. He still glances at the photos of the *mahamana*s (*maha* = great; *mana* = mind). He still hums, and sometimes, my mother intercepts him to put a few drops of *charana-amrta* or sandalwood on his lips.

The morning ritual to fill the *indriyas* with something sweet before the world takes over is a conscious act of allegiance to our perceptive self. Āyurveda tells us that the intake of positive energy at the beginning of the day will set the tone for what the universe will bring later and how we will receive it.

Sugandha (*su* = prefix in Sanskrit meaning good, excellent, virtuous and beautiful; *gandha* = smell) is a sweet, fragrant smell, in allegiance to the element of earth. In the morning, we can smell a flower, burning incense or even sweet fresh air from the trees or mountains. In India, most homes either keep sticks of *agarbatti*/ incense, perfume or flowers.

Sumukha (*mukh* = mouth; opening) gives us something sweet to taste. It can be a small piece of fruit, a piece of rock sugar or a sweet or fragrant leaf. Tulsi leaves are commonly put on the tongue first thing in the morning for *sumukha*, in allegiance to the element of water.

Sudriśti (*driś* = sight) is something pleasant to see. It can be the mountains outside your window or a beautiful forest or a baby sleeping next to you. It can be the people you love. Anything beautiful that pleases the eyes and inspires the mind is a tribute to the element of fire.

Sukatha (*katha* = utterance) gives the voice first use by passing wind through the vocal cords for speaking virtuous words, as an allegiance to the element of air. One can recite a poem, a verse or a sacred prayer. Mantras are commonly recited if they are sweet.

Sushabda (*shabd* = sound in Sanskrit) passes waves through the ethers to our ears, in allegiance to the element of space. People invoke early morning instrumental music, the *shankh*, a melodious voice or a gentle hum that pleases the ear.

If an attractive, beautiful-minded person greets you with fragrant flowers, singing in a melodious voice, and then speaks some beautiful words to you and offers you a bite of something clean, sweet and fresh, your day is set.

But for the hurried urban, Westernized person on the go, who still wants to complete the rituals of the early morning *dinacharya*, for one-stop efficiency, keep rock sugar on the altar, next to incense, a beautiful picture of a deity, clean water and a book of mantras.

> ❧ Engage each of the five senses with something pleasant in the morning, such as incense, flowers, a picture of a deity, clean water, recitation of mantras and rock sugar.

Many early morning cultural rituals fulfil this routine of invoking the five senses without people being consciously aware of their origin. Āyurveda tells us we may look at our parents, elders or clean priests; we may find a cow or look at water. We may gaze at the sacred fire or look at gold, ghee or the sun as early morning starters. These are also considered auspicious, primarily because they fill the mind with peace and happiness.

The modern world has adapted these rituals with its own product version. In the urban modern world, we see heavy marketing to encourage people to begin the day with deodorant to feel smooth and smell fresh, then douse themselves with alcohol-based perfumes and fragrant hair sprays and gels. There is a strong preference for a morning cup of coffee. People gaze at beautiful paintings of nature on their walls, listen to music on their electronic digitized players and rush off into the world.

Āyurveda asks you to stop and be aware of your senses, to consciously begin the day by choosing nature and sacred relationships to fill your *indriyas*, as you start your day.

❧

~ • 11 • ~

Framing the Day

Even at this stage of life, enduring post-stroke paralysis, my father is steadfast in his daily routine, as much of it as he can do. After his morning predawn cup of tea and meditation, he hobbles with his cane up to the toilet, where he urinates, empties his bowels, washes his hands, cleans his dentures and teeth, scrapes his tongue and clips his facial hair, all with one hand. He slowly oils his face, nose, ears and puts ghee on his eyes. He then applies oil that has been warmed in a metal bowl over hot water in the sink on his body. In winter, my mother brings him oil warmed on the stove and turns on the bathroom heater. He then goes into the shower and completes his morning cleansing routine with a look in the mirror before he hobbles out and looks at the photos of Einstein, Tagore and Vivekananda hanging in the house.

My father's routine has kept many parts of him very healthy. At the age of seventy-five, he has a nearly perfect physique, no midriff fat and strong, taut muscles on the right side of his body that still sense and move. The stroke did not take the toll on him that it does on most Americans that survive such traumas. His *dinacharya* has oriented him towards choices that support him despite some level of Western diet and lifestyle. His image of himself is strongly reflected in his choices. He still has a strong desire to dress in his nice trousers and sweaters and wear his fine shirts and rings. His closet is still kept perfectly, with perfectly spaced wooden hangers, expensive ties hanging precisely, his wing-tipped shoes, handkerchiefs and cuff links neatly assembled next to his kurtas, pyjamas and flawless woollen shawls. When we dress him for a formal occasion, he enjoys it and does not want to undress at the end of the day. But he is no longer the strong man he was. He is a child in an old man's body. I wonder what he sees when he looks in the mirror.

Āyurveda tells us to finish our early-morning routine by looking at our own reflection. It is a check to make sure that we set up our physical appearance and approve of how we are presenting ourselves to the world. What others will see is about their own *indriya*s, but we should be happy with our own appearance and how we reflect our state of health and happiness. When we are *beauty-full* to ourselves, we have more confidence and live with our hearts more open to the bounty of the universe.

In the days before mirrors, we looked into a pond or a still water body. Āyurveda warned not to lean into a river, and not look at one's reflection in a well. It advised that we look at ourselves in sacred, clean reflections in the morning, in a brook or in a pot of water or ghee, after bathing and before prayers.

- Finish your early morning routine by observing your reflection after meditation.
- Note whether you are happy and satisfied with your appearance.

❧

pranamya devān vrddhāmscha mangalāshtaśatam śūbham |
śrnvan kāñchanavinya*stam sarpih paśyodanantaram* ||*23*||

After gods and elders are worshipped, the 108 auspicious names of God should be repeated while the person looks at his/her own image in a golden vessel filled with ghee.

Astānga Samgraha of Vāgbhata,
Sūtra-sthāna; chapter 3, sloka 23

❧

True beauty is more than skin deep. Āyurveda emphasizes that skin is a reflection of the deeper layers of the body's tissues and of the digestive *agni*. It emphasizes the importance of inner cleanliness, good nutrition and proper functioning of the digestive *agni*. When the body is in a state of perfect flow and function, it exudes an energy known as *ojas* that is alluring, attractive and unforgettable.

Āyurveda also places emphasis on reflecting inner calm and goodness as part of outer beauty. The forty-three muscles of the face can often tell people what is really going on inside. Scientists, especially Dr Paul Ekman, have found that there are seven emotions that present very clear facial signals: surprise, happiness, disgust, contempt, sadness, fear and anger. Research shows that when a person arranges his/her face into a certain expression, he/she will actually feel the corresponding emotion. Emotions work from the outside inward and also from the inside outward. When we make certain facial movements, they seem to turn on the corresponding physical sensations for particular emotions. Therefore, perfect calm and happiness that is reflected on a symmetric face actually corresponds to peace inside. Perceptive people sense these micro-expressions in others, and that is why good businessmen will insist on meeting in person for important discussions and signing of important documents.

Instinctively, we judge people based on their facial expressions. When a face is kept neatly, it reflects good inner health. A symmetric face is also considered a reflection of balance and a scientific element of identifying beauty. Perfectly aligned faces are rare, but they reflect that something right happened, some perfection has remained. Another reflection of beauty is the observable hygiene of the sense organs. When the five senses are clean and functioning optimally, the face is open, harmoniously ready to receive and thus attractive. Though we know that excretions are a normal part of eyes, ears, nose and mouth, somehow we do not want to see substances leaking out from the orifices. When we check our reflection in the mirror, we make sure that all of these normal substances have been cleaned away, lest they give a subtle signal about cleanliness we did not intend to deliver.

The Early Morning Routine: Practical

The practical reality of adopting a steady early-morning routine aligned with Āyurvedic principles requires that you first assess where you are. Do you already do five or six of the rituals? Or are you woefully disorganized in the morning? The way to start is around the morning ablutions, as going to the bathroom is usually an act of nature. As you rise in the morning, adopt one ritual you have read that appeals to you and adopt it. Work on it every day until it becomes a loved and adherent part of your morning schedule. Then add another ritual, doing it as correctly as it seems to be prescribed. Make adjustments. Read. Alter your bathroom set-up, your closet or night table.

Once you have adopted most of the rituals, you will find yourself changing. I am not yet sure how this happens or when the neurobiology behind it will be revealed. But I have seen it in hundreds of patients. They become happier. They become healthier. They avert disease, and they cure small health problems that were recurrent. Some cure their big health issues. There is something about the early-morning routine that cleans the senses, aligns the body with the forces of nature and realigns it with health.

When the rituals have been adopted, they take about 11 minutes to do at a normal pace. If one rises around an hour-and-a-half before dawn and lies still, one will hear one's belly conveying how it is, what it wants and some other unexpected information from the gut instinct that is inside each of us. Then bend fully down, touch the ground with the hands and say a prayer before stepping onto the earth. Take a small sip of water from the right palm, as the practice of *ācamana* describes. Then head towards the toilet, perhaps putting water on to boil if there is time. If you are not feeling the urge to go, do some exercise to contract your abdominal muscles. After clearing the bladder and bowels, wash the hands well. Then wash the face, splash cold water on the eyes, inhale a bit of water into each nostril and expel it completely, and swish some water in the mouth. Clean the teeth next, using an appropriate brush or stick and appropriate herbs, powders or dentrifice. Begin with the bottom teeth first; brush behind the teeth on top, and in the front, as well as along the gum line in front and the back. Rinse the mouth, then scrape the tongue using 3–4 long movements from the back of the tongue towards the front and then rinse the mouth again.

As you walk out of the washing area, look at an auspicious object and some photos of loved ones that make your heart warm. Light a candle or look at the sun safely if it has come up. Light some incense or smell something pleasant. Say an inspiring prayer. Hum a mantra or tune. Put a fresh leaf of tulsi on your tongue. Look in the mirror and head for the kitchen to sip your hot water as you begin your day.

❧

Part II:
Opening the Five Senses

As I listen to the drone of a pithy, monotonous Āyurvedic doctor on a teleconference about *dinacharya*, I look into some yawning half-filled boxes in the hallway of our grand house. I try to pay attention to him preaching routines of a healthy daily life, but all I can do is smirk, recalling my father bouncing at the foot of my bed until I awoke for the day's lesson on how to live. When I finally rose and shared those predawn hours, I was keenly aware of our freedom, oblivious to time and the demands of others. Our senses opened to the day and soared into the ethers as we discussed life.

Once the sky lit up though, my father would disappear upstairs. He would close the door to start his 'routine'. As a child, I wondered what that routine was. Surely, he did not sit in the bathroom for an hour. Yet, when he emerged from the locked humid room, un-shirted, with wet hair and his sacred thread over his left shoulder, ready to sit in the prayer room, it seemed that all he had done was shower. It perplexed me as I considered our simple childlike preparations of brushing teeth and combing. I would sneak into his bathroom, peering into the bowls and vessels remaining after he departed, comparing the instruments of his morning routine with their vivid colours and odours.

By the age of ten, when my father disappeared upstairs, I knew my day was also beginning, as a school-prompted morning rush pierced our sacred bubble of protected time. My bathroom chores were prompt and orderly—morning ablutions and washing the face, eyes, nose, mouth, teeth and tongue. Wherever we lived, my mother installed a full set of tools in the medicine cabinet for the morning routine: toothpaste, toothpowder, different colours and shapes of brushes, combs, scrapers, spoons, soaps, floss and oil.

But there were a few boxes in the side closet for special routines and alternatives. These would be introduced for a few days for one of us when my mother instructed a special routine prompted by a cold, flu, rash or infection. We would witness my mother administer an oil, a salve or a powder. Over years, my life was ingrained with the smells and flavours of these special routines for cleaning our eyes, ears, nose and mouth.

❧

Āyurveda separately emphasizes clean senses in its definitions of a healthy being. Unlike other holistic systems that discuss the Being as body, mind and sometimes the soul, which Descartes removed from the domain of medicine in 1648, Āyurvedic philosophy also focuses on a fourth component, the *indriyas* as the interactive tool connecting the outer world and our inner purpose for living.

Jñana-indriyas (*jñana* = wisdom in Sanskrit) are the five sensory organs, *karma-indriyas* (*karma* = action) are the five motor organs, and *manas* is the organ for sensing the soul and connecting it to the language of the senses. Together, these eleven organs act to help the soul journey around in the material world on its path of discovery and healing.

Humans have five sense organs that interact with the five master elements on the planet. These five elements are indivisible for living things and are different from the elements in the chemical periodic table. Called *panchamahabhuta*s (*pancha* = five; *maha* = great), *bhuta* literally means that derived from a non-material energetic being. These energies, from most subtle to most material, are space, air, fire, water and earth.

Sometimes called ether (think of ethereal), space is the physical absence of molecules and represents the potential for being filled by material. Its medium or *tanmatra* is sound. *Tanmatra* is the subtle energy whose movement allows our consciousness to sense and thereby create an interpretation with which the body can interact. When space moves, we perceive sound. Without the harmony of sound, we could not listen. The *jñana-indriya* is the organ of sound or the eardrum and inner ear architecture and mechanics.

Air is the element that is made of transparent molecules. Without the presence of these lightly packed, fast-moving molecules, we would not be able to detect movement. The *tanmatra* of air is touch. Air allows us to sense both sound and touch. When air moves, we are able to perceive feeling. Modern science says we perceive through sensory receptors of four main types—hot/cold, pressure, pain and position. Other animals, especially fish, have a sixth sense in electroreceptors, which detect electric fields, salinity and temperature gradients. The *jñana-indriya* is the organ of our skin.

Fire is the element of heat and earth. Its *tanmatra* is form, which we perceive as vision through the *jñana-indriya* of the eye. Fire interacts with sound, touch and vision. The movement of subtle fire is known as light, without which we could not see form or colour.

Water is the predominant element on earth. It is the solvent, solution and crystal in which life is made. Its *tanmatra* is taste. Water interacts with sound, touch, vision and taste. Only when water moves and interacts with other elements are we able to perceive different tastes. The taste buds are the *jñana-indriya.* Containing gustatory receptors, these sit predominantly on our tongue and in our stomach. If you dry your tongue completely, and then run sugar or salt across your tongue, you will not be able to taste anything.

Earth is the heaviest element on the planet. It has many forms and characteristics, including inorganic metals and rocks and organic wood and plants. It provides structure and stability to everything in the material world. Its *tanmatra* is odour. Earth interacts with sound, touch, vision, taste and smell. When the earth moves, it can interact with our organs of smell, called olfactory receptors, which are in the nose and tongue, and activate the smell receptors. Without the particles and density of earth, we would not be able to trigger our smell receptors.

These five elements convey subtle properties of energy translating into matter. Our five sense organs pick up the subtle energies and matter, and translate them into our consciousness through forms we can perceive enough to identify. Light, sound and invisible chemicals become sound, touch, form, taste and smell.

Self-control of the sense organs is said to be the greatest promoter of delight and the ability to be content. The discipline of yoga and the study of *adhyatmika* both address the yoking of the mind, with its infinite possibilities and quick movement. The sense organs, the five *gyan-indriyas*, interface our mind and soul with the world. Overstimulation of the sense organs leads to addictions, uncompensated desires and the *ripu* or trappings of the mind. Understimulation leads to withdrawal, depression, lack of connection and hopelessness from lack of experience. Aberrant stimulations lead to perverted thoughts that make us see the world in patterns that are not harmonious with the way nature flows. Thus, self-control allows us to engage our hearing, touching/feeling, sight, smell and taste with the world around us and enjoy the balance that is nature. This attunement to harmony provides delight and contentment that is often translated as happiness.

khādīnyātmā manaḥ kālō diśaśca dravyasaṅgrahaḥ |
sēndriyaṁ cētanaṁ dravyaṁ, nirindriyamacētanam ||*48*||

The five elements (*prthvi, ap, tejas, vayu* and *akasa*), soul, mind, time and space constitute physical matter, creating the material world and the body. A system or collection of matter with sense and motor organs can be sentient, while one devoid of them is insentient.

Caraka Samhita,
Sūtra-sthāna; chapter 1, sloka 48

Āyurveda spends considerable energy advising how to keep the five senses and the mind clean. It reminds us to re-invigorate and open them so that we can take in the world. Rather than relegate them to an ENT doctor when a problem arises, Āyurveda teaches us how to keep health care in the self-empowered domain, as we are often the only ones that can detect when a disturbance in our senses has occurred. It advises us to clean our senses each morning, and then periodically, so that we can engage with our environment, actively counselling, communicating and forming relationships through eye contact, active listening and knowledge of how to talk to and touch another person appropriately.

Part II:

Opening the Five Senses

~ • 12 • ~

Cleaning the Senses: The Eyes

Early every morning since before my birth, my mother goes to greet the sun. In every house, every land, she would find him—either from the verandah, atop the roof or outside on the grounds, yard or driveway. She would utter the mantra that greets the sun,

om jaba-kusum shanka-shan kashyapeyam
maha-dhyutim dhanta-warim sarvo-papagna
pranatoshmi diva-karam ||

Salutations to that, red as a hibiscus flower turning to white, pure as the saint Kashyapa,

To that which is grand in shimmering brightness; which takes darkness away and annihilates all sins

I give pranam to He who creates the day.

Surya Pranam/Surya Namaskar

She would look directly at the rising sun if it was still touching the earth, and then she would continue her day. Once, my sister the NASA astrophysicist, counselled her on the danger of looking directly at the sun. She explained that the sun's heat, brightness and ability to burn a hole into the retina could blind a person. My mother listened to her admonitions, blinked, paused and remained silent. That evening, I watched her ask the sun for forgiveness as she waited until it touched the earth, and again she uttered her mantra.

For my mother and hundreds of millions of Indians who have greeted the sun this way without going blind, *trāṭaka* is a way of life. In Sanskrit, the practice of *trāṭaka* means to gaze fixedly and is used to induce meditation and *sthira* (stillness) by concentrating on a single point. As a technique of yoga used to develop awareness, attention and focus, it strengthens the eyes and stimulates the *ājnā* chakra or third eye.

There are three phases to *trāṭaka* practice. The first phase involves stilling the voluntary movements of the eyes. Fix your gaze on a non-moving object and try to hold a steady gaze for a minute or more. In this first phase, the mind will wander, and the eyes will want to move. When a thought or feeling arises, notice it and then let it go. Keep staring. After a few seconds, the eyes will want to close. Keep them open. When they begin to water, close them gently, allowing the heat and emotions to release with the tears. Once you can stare for 1 minute, move on to the second phase.

In the second phase, stare intently at a live candle flame. Watch it and let the eyes become still as the flicker continues to move. Transcend the movement and keep the eyes open until they water, then close them gently, allowing the heat and emotions to release with the tears. With the eyes closed, hold the after-image of the candle for as long as you can.

In the third phase, you must greet the sun as it rises. You may put ghee on the eyes before starting. Find the sun while the globe is still red or deep orange and still touching the horizon. Stare into the sun only if it does not hurt and keep the eyes as still as possible. Depending on where you are, the sun will move quite fast and you will only have an interval of 10–15 minutes to do your *trāṭaka* practice in the morning and evening. Once it stops touching the horizon, you should NOT do *trāṭaka* with the sun. Use a candle instead.

Practice *trāṭaka* in the following three phases:

- First Phase: Fix your gaze on a non-moving object and try to hold it for a minute or more. When a thought or feeling arises, notice it and then let it go. When the eyes want to close, keep them open. When they begin to water, close them gently, allowing the heat and emotions to release with the tears. Once you can stare for 1 minute, move on to the second phase.
- Second Phase: Stare intently at a live candle flame. Watch it and let the eyes become still as the flicker continues to move. Transcend the movement and keep the eyes open until they water, then close them gently, allowing the heat and emotions to release with the tears. With the eyes closed, hold the after-image of the candle for as long as you can.
- Third Phase: Greet the sun as it rises. You may put ghee on the eyes before starting. Look at the sun only when it is red or deep orange, and still touching the horizon. Stare into the sun only if it does not hurt and keep the eyes as still as possible. You will only have an interval of 10–15 minutes to do your *trāṭaka* practice in the morning and evening. Once it stops touching the horizon, you should NOT do *trāṭaka* with the sun. Use a candle instead.

❧

The eyes are essentially extensions of the fat blobs that compose our brain and nervous system. The nerves are essentially encased in fat, and the eyes are made of the same tissue and directly connected, from the deepest core of the brain, shielded in skull bone for protection as it emerges outward from the head as probes for the body. The eyes are modified nerves that capture energy in the form of light and sometimes heat. This anatomy is amazingly similar in most animals.

The human eye has three fluid compartments, surrounded by fat on all sides of its ball shape. Under the thick, clear outside protein shield of the eye, called the cornea, the first fluid compartment is filled with aqueous humour—the anterior chamber—and covers the coloured muscles of the round iris. Through the narrow opening of the iris, known as the pupil, is the second compartment—called the posterior chamber. Problems in this area, especially increases in pressure, cause glaucoma. Behind a thin film at the back of this space is the chamber holding the aqueous humour, a watery fluid that is responsible for hydration and circulation to the eye. Behind it is a large cavity known as the vitreous body or vitreous humour, which gives shape to the eye and lubricates the nerves that lie at the back of the eye and connect it to the brain.

When we see, the light that enters the anterior chamber shoots back through the vitreous humour and lands on the back of the eye in an area that has light receptors to detect colour or black/white. These receptors send the information directly to many areas of the brain, instantaneously interpreting a hundred things and making it known that we saw something.

The eyes perceive how far away something is and how thick it is, by integrating slightly different angles of light from each eye, bouncing off the same object. The eyes also detect and distinguish colour, contrast and amount of light, see in the night, track movements, focus on objects both near and far away, and create balance through other information from the body about where it is in relation to other objects. Some say the eye can only see those wavelengths of light in the visual spectrum, from the edge of ultraviolet light—at 390 nanometers in the violet range—to 780 nanometers in the deep red range, at the edge of infrared light. Others say that some people can sense even in the infrared light range or see hazes that are beyond 780nm, which are visible to animals such as bees, dogs, cats, cattle, reindeer, hedgehogs, bats, ferrets and okapis.

Despite all the details known about the neuroscience of the eye, conventional medicine has not been able to use billions of funded dollars to recover lost vision. Today, blindness due to diabetic retinopathy, cataracts and macular degeneration are considered incurable by modern medicine. Infections such as conjunctivitis and blepharitis are treated with steroids and antibiotics, and complications from eye surgeries, contact lenses and lens implants continue.

Because fat melts more easily than other tissues, and nerve tissues are composed of special fats that are especially sensitive to heat, it is better not to overheat the eyes, which are actually modified nerves. This is why Āyurveda suggests cool water for the eyes every morning.

Ancient Āyurveda gave us tools to keep the eyes healthy through the toils of the day, emphasizing the prevention of disease through daily maintenance and periodic rituals that strengthen the eyes. The first was washing the eyes with cold water in the early-morning routine, keeping solid and stable the oils and fat that comprise the eyes.

Each night before bed, I put ghee into my eyes for routine cleansing and as my favourite beauty ritual. Starting on the eyelids of both eyes, I rub clean ghee into the skin, then to the margin of the lids, until ghee seeps into the space and covers the eyeball. When things look hazy, it means enough ghee has penetrated.

Used to clean the eyes, ghee is cooling in nature according to Āyurveda and has the same fats that the human body requires for its cells and functioning of its tissues. Most patients who use ghee regularly have told me they feel their eyes look more sharp, that the whites look cleaner and that they feel less fear of putting things into their eyes after using ghee for a few nights.

While it is safe, the practice is foreign to most modern-day, westernized people and thus, this practice is best done the first time by watching and then practising on others before trying on your own.

- Splash cold water on the eyes each morning.
- Once you have carefully observed someone apply ghee, follow these steps yourself:
  - Apply it before going to bed.
  - Begin with the eyelids of both eyes, rubbing clean ghee into the skin.
  - Then extend to the margin of the lids, until ghee seeps into the space and covers the eyeball.
  - When things look hazy, it means enough ghee has penetrated.

According to Āyurveda, the eyes, while oily and fatty in nature, are dominated by functions of *vāta* and *pitta*. *Vāta* is the reflection of the quality of movement, and *pitta* is the reflection of the theme of transformation.

Fire and water are sharp, fiery and acidic. The theme underlying these qualities is transformation and called *pitta*. Fire and water do not mix and seem to be an impossible combination. Put a potato in fire and it will char to ash; in water, it will sit and spoil. But put it in water in a vessel on top of fire, between the two elements, and working together, they transform the potato into a delicious, edible item.

This transformation also occurs in the eye. The eye transforms light that reflects off things in our environment, which makes its way through the oily balls filled with water to the back of the eye, into information about objects, calling it vision. Thus, heat is constantly produced by the photons coming into the eye.

Sankhya philosophy espouses that we have our five senses to interact with the physical world. Fire, with its light, brightness and heat is sensed primarily through our eyes, though each of our five senses also detect aspects of fire through touch and sound, and through smell and taste indirectly.

In the body, the theme of transformation oversees a multitude of vital functions and the associated structures that are needed to fulfil those functions: the digestive portions of the gut, the biotransformation enzymes of the liver, the various bits of information conveyed by the skin and the fiery will of the mind/soul that is sometimes called self-determination.

It follows that diseases in these areas disturb the theme of transformation and therefore disturb the balance of *pitta* in the body. The body requires the *pitta* to be balanced for healthy transformation to take place.

When the eyes have too much sharpness, fire and acidity, they are *pitta*-dominated. The result is poor quality of transformation. The heat of fire and the sharpness create hot, dry eyes that burn and tingle as the oily tissues dry out. The dryness and burning lead to itching and inflammation, which present as redness, swelling, pain and sensation of heat. Āyurveda interpreted these signs and symptoms as a whole with the term *pitta*. In the eyes, it is called *alochaka pitta*.

The wise men that gathered the ancient knowledge of Āyurveda had amazing perception and excellent sight. They were able to discern subtle properties of plants, animals and foods, categorize them and predict what would happen if substances were combined. In their wisdom, they knew that care of the eyes was dependent on renewal, regular cleansing and flushing, and remoistening.

A regular ritual of many yogis is to apply raw honey to their eyes once in 3 weeks, just before bedtime. Raw honey, known as *madhu* or *maksika* in Sanskrit, is sweet and astringent. According to ancient chemistry, honey has scraping properties to remove grime and oil but is gentle and effective. Perhaps due to salivary enzymes of the bee mixed with digested pollen, it is drying and cleansing as it promotes digestion of toxins.

The first time is the scariest, so it is best to be guided by a seasoned user. Place one drop of clean honey on a clean finger pad, then guide the finger towards the eye. Create a pocket opening at the eye's bottom lid by pulling the under-eye skin downward. Place the drop of honey into the pocket and gently close the eyes while breathing deeply. Within 10 seconds, a deep burning and ache will emerge. It is not a sharp pain, but it will shake a few people. Breathe deeply. The eyes will sting and burn for a few seconds, followed by a tangible sense of different fluids in the eyes. Slowly, a heat will emerge from within the eye, like a snake coalescing then winding its way outward. A feeling of something emerging will occur within half a minute. Heavy tears will well up and fall, and then the eyes will feel light and fresh and clean. The first time, my patients curse my name and scream, then sing praises when the purification is over. Thus is the nature of cleansing.

If you are putting honey in the eyes for the first time, follow these steps under the guidance of an experienced user:

- Place one drop of clean honey on a clean finger pad and then guide the finger towards the eye.
- Create a pocket opening at the lid by pulling the under-eye skin downward.
- Place the drop of honey into the pocket and gently close the eyes while breathing deeply.

Early one morning, an old patient called me suddenly with news that his nephew had been hit near the eye socket with a cricket ball. With his vision compromised, bleeding and pain, he had been rushed to the hospital. The physician had examined him and declared that his vision in one part of his right eye was lost and diminished in another. Bleeding indicated detachment of the retina. The young man was advised to apply a patch, take some pain killers and rest until the wound healed.

Āyurveda reminds us that oils have curative powers. The body is *sheeta, snigdha* and *agneya*, which means that by nature, it is cool, moisture-adherent and transformative like fire. In times of distress, we may turn to these properties to aid healing. Remembering this principle, combined with the knowledge of anatomy, the young man was asked if he wanted to try *netra basti*, also called *netra tarpana*. Three of his family agreed to learn the treatment that could work if properly prepared and applied meticulously for 7 days. Willing to undertake the challenge, materials were gathered quickly: ghee, *urad* flour, clean water, gauze, clean bowls and a spoon. Within three hours of the injury, the treatment was begun.

Laying the patient comfortably on his back, a hot washcloth was used to apply steam to his forehead, temples, cheeks and nose. The purpose was to heat the skin and improve circulation around the eyes and sinuses, and to comfort him. Then, the head was tilted back slightly so that the eye sockets faced the sky. A round sticky doughnut was created from *urad* flour and clean water, and placed around the eye socket, creating a wall sealed to the skin under the eyebrows, along the nose and under the eyes. Into this pool, cool liquid ghee was poured by slowing squeezing a gauze that had been dipped into a bowl. The ghee was filled to the edge of the pool that had been created in the centre of the doughnut. After some time, he slowly opened his eye. On one side, his field of vision was still intact, and he could look through the yellow liquid, slightly heavy on his orbit. The rest of his vision was dark.

This treatment was done twice a day for 7 days with the help of two members of his family. On the fourth day, his mother informed me that the young man had woken up seeing more from his right eye and able to move it freely. I was adamant they should continue for 7 days before assessment. On the seventh evening, his vision had returned fully but was cloudy. They offered to continue for another week and I agreed.

The family avoided me after the first month. Much later, I learnt that his vision was tested by the same ophthalmologist at the same hospital and was found to be normal. They had rejoiced and felt it unnecessary to contact the 'ghee doctor'. The real doctor who had pronounced him blind earlier did not ask too many questions but was happy to take payment for his testing. There was a lot of fear from this simple family about payment to me, since they had spent so much for the doctor. I took one rupee, because vision is priceless. What I learnt from this young man about *netra basti* could not be repaid with money.

Netra basti is used for a variety of conditions, including chronic dry eyes, poor vision, inflamed eyes, scratched corneas and degenerative conditions of the eye. Each case must be handled individually, in the context of fire in the person's body, stability and transformative power vs. charring nature of the fire.

In my emergency kit, I keep a glass bottle of *mahatriphala ghrit*. *Ghrit* is the Sanskrit term for ghee with medicinal herbs cooked into it. *Mahatriphala* is a combination of over a dozen herbs that calm the heat and dryness of *vāta* and *pitta* that imbalance the eyes. For millennia, it has been used to cleanse the eyes, treat burning and itching, and revive the eyes after illnesses, inflammation, infection, surgery and chronic irritation. Āyurvedic physicians sometimes prescribe these edible herbs to be cooked in ghee and ingested with *triphala kwath* (decoction). Contrary to conventional beliefs, the older the ghee, the more medicinal it becomes.

Mahatriphala ghrit is a dangerous compound, not because of its efficacy, safety or non-toxicity, but only because it is simple and therefore, threatens the medical perception that eyes should only be treated by doctors. It is one of the compounds that underscores the problems of preconceived bias of conventional medical researchers against traditional medicines and self-care.

Firstly, it is a poly-herbal substance. Conventional doctors will ask which compound is the effective one because they are trained to believe that only one chemical can be the target drug in a scenario. They will ponder over the quagmire of problems in a compound that has hundreds, indeed thousands, of unknown chemicals. It is difficult for them to conceive that the overall efficacy of a drug can be due to many interdependent factors that create an overall effect.

Secondly, the compound is being put into the eyes. People are wary of anything eye-bound and wonder about toxicity to the eye.

In fact, hundreds of thousands of people have used *mahatriphala ghrit* and reported improvements. It is legal to use under Indian law, under Section 3a of the Drugs and Cosmetics Act, as a classical Āyurvedic medicine listed and described in detail in classical Āyurvedic texts. But it is still reluctantly approached by doctors both in India as well as around the world.

Thirdly, ghee has been vilified, beginning with an article in *The Lancet*, a prestigious medical journal, in September 1987. Using ghee not made by Āyurvedic standards, the authors made waves by linking atherosclerosis with cholesterol oxides found in ghee. They created an impression of the dangers of ghee by outlining risk factors for heart disease, with subsequent articles about ghee, warning patients about diabetes, high cholesterol and high blood pressure. People today talk of the excessive fat in ghee, which indeed contains over 60 per cent saturated fat and 8 mg of cholesterol per teaspoon, not acknowledging the good fat to bad fat ratio that differs across preparations of ghee. Indeed, conventional medicine has also shown that the body needs 'good fats' and that some cholesterol-lowering agents deplete the body of fats that can lead to brain deterioration, since the brain contains 25 percent of the body's cholesterol. Science has now also shown that information is transmitted to the brain via little fat droplets that travel in a network along the nerve cells, called the inter-axon network, and not only through the blood, as previously thought.

But while Āyurveda recommends ghee as one of the best substances for nourishing the body, strengthening tissues and aiding metabolism, it also warns that ghee should not be used when digestion is poor and toxins are high, as the fat will not melt properly and clog the micro-channels of the body, hampering movement and flow. Just as oil on a strong fire will increase the fire, the same oil on a weak fire will put it out. Understanding how much oil to pour into a fire is similar to understanding how much ghee a person can consume. There is no mention of such calculations of the body's metabolic strength in most of the research studies on ghee, and so it is vilified.

However, popular use often outsmarts all the concern that scientists have when they lack evidence. A huge upsurge of use began in 2005, when several classical Āyurvedic formulas became popular with the endorsement of Baba Ramdev on television and the Internet. People starting using ghee on their own, rubbing it into their eyes every night and reporting their own clinical results. As expected, it has been safe and not linked with any toxicity or blindness.

In the heart of south India, Āyurvedic formulas using combinations of herbs are in abundance, especially in the hot tropical climate of Kerala. *Elaneer kuzhambu* is an elixir made specially for cleaning wounds and ulcerations of the eye, cataracts and conjunctivitis—conditions associated with *pitta* and *kapha*. It is not to be used in *vāta* disorders of the eye, which manifest as dryness, sharp pain or fear of being touched in the eye.

The thick liquid has nine components, all of which are used in other Āyurvedic formulas for eye conditions, including the cleansing super-trio of *triphala*: *amalaki* the superfood, *haritaki* the cleanser and *bibhitaki* the melter. It also contains honey, coconut water, camphor and liquorice. Ingredients promoting eye health are called *caksusya* in Sanskrit. Most are light, stimulating digestion and transformation of any impurities that may be irritating or inflaming the eyes.

This viscous and concentrated liquid is applied in the soft light of late evening as eye drops or eyeliner to the bottom lid margin, starting from the inner lid, moving outward toward the temple, and then closing the eye and rolling the eyeball to spread the thick liquid through the sclera or mucous covering the eyeball. The eyes will tear and if desired, may be washed with *triphala* powder mixed in water and filtered to make an eyewash. Else, drying the tears, resting the eyes completely and then sleeping soon after is advised.

In one of the workshops teaching *dinacharya*, we offered health professionals the chance to volunteer and experience *elaneer kuzhambu*. One began to weep and after a few minutes, to howl. She excused herself and emerged half an hour later, sharing with the group the clearing she had experienced, as images from her past reappeared before her eyes before melting away with the elixir. The surreal experience stayed with her for weeks, and she changed her life and relationships according to the powerful visions she had watched melt before her. She was not alone. There were several students who had experienced profound cleansing, which revealed a sense of coolness in the eyes, sharper vision and a feeling of lightness as well as an unexpected emotional cleansing. Over the years, I have added this bottle to my recommendations for weekly beauty treatments, especially for actors and people who wear a lot of eye make-up or spend a lot of time in front of the computer screen.

To use *elaneer kuzhambu*, follow these instructions:

- Apply this liquid eye drop during the soft light of late evening to the bottom lid margin.
- Start from the inner lid and move outward toward the temple. Then close the eye and roll the eyeball to spread the thick liquid through the sclera, the mucous covering the eyeball.
- Wash away tears with *triphala* powder mixed in water and filtered to make an eyewash. Else, dry the tears and rest the eyes completely.

Eyeliners have been used through the ages. Now they come in a spectrum of colours and application types: pencils, liquids, cakes and tubes with brushes. Originally called *anjana* in Sanskrit, the eyeliner was designed as a way of applying medicinal herbs to the eyes to clean, cool and purify them regularly. It was also conceived that negative energies, called *nazar* in many cultures from Paris to Tokyo, could penetrate the eyes and thus the soul. *Anjana* was also thought to prevent these evil spirits from penetrating the eyes.

Anjana, or kohl, was made by cooking herbs known to be good for the eyes, such as *amalaki*, *haritaki* or berberry, on an iron griddle until they burned to ash. A drop of oil was added to the fine blackened grit, which was cooled and stored in clean jars, and applied every day with a clean stick or finger pad to the margin of the bottom eyelid, especially to children's eyes, to prevent infections.

Collyrium derives from a Greek term *kollurion*, meaning poultice, and is the antique term for liquids, gels or gritty salves used to cleanse the eye. In the Western world, herbs such as rose, eyebright and fennel were used. In Āyurveda, metals are sometimes used due to their keen ability to be toxic to bacteria. In modern-day medicine, silver nitrate gel is still applied to newborn eyes in many hospitals to kill deadly bacteria, such as the one that causes gonorrhoea, which may penetrate the eyes during its passage through the vaginal canal.

Modern eyeliners made by commercial giants use heavy metals as preservatives for lengthening shelf life and petroleum-based chemicals; they no longer use medicinal herbs for the eye. Their use of mercury or lead is exempted by the drugs and cosmetics laws of most countries. Sharing applicators is not encouraged but is common.

Yoga has become a craze in the US. Not only is it a lucrative business that requires very little financial investment, but the yoga teacher also benefits from watching students improve their lives. After much prodding, I attended a class of a self-proclaimed-famous yogi who claimed he had taught yoga at the White House and to an armful of dignitaries. His special yoga was face yoga, a new popular craze because of its effectiveness on beauty. The exercises focus on the anatomy and physiology of facial muscles and the cranial nerves that regulate the brain's control of the face.

In a programmed and smooth flow, the yogi led us through a sequence of exercises for the face. He began with the forehead, then moved on to the temples, ears, eyes, cheeks, nose, mouth and finally, to the neck. The session lasted 45 minutes, and people were encouraged to repeat the exercises each morning in front of the mirror or in a meditative state on a yoga mat.

Eye yoga is very similar to examinations doctors use to test the functions of the cranial nerves (III, IV and VI) in and around the eyes. The patient is instructed to look near then far, move the eyes up then down, left then right, dart diagonally left-to-right then diagonally right-to-left, make semicircles clockwise then counterclockwise, and finally, the eyelids are opened wide then pressed shut. These exercises when combined with a meditative state are thought to tone the muscles around the eye and reconnect the skin with the muscles and layers underneath.

Around the age of seven, when I was in fourth grade, I began rubbing my eyes because there was a haze around people when I looked at them. Other objects were fairly clear. My sister, whom I mimicked and followed like a chicken behind a hen, complained of fuzziness and with her prompts, I recalled that sometimes the chalkboard was not sharp as well. Advised by the school teachers, my father had us taken to a doctor. My first pair of eyeglasses were tiny, oblong, lake-blue plastic frames that I detested. The only thing that made them bearable was that my sister got a similar pair.

They arrived soon after we landed in the US and were a sign that the country would improve our third-world lives by giving us clearer vision. But somehow I felt that the glasses put a filter between me and the world. It was as though I had to see the falsehoods in front of me as truth just because they appeared sharp. What I saw clearly, as the only brown girl in my class at school in Omaha, was a land filled with racism, despite cries of freedom and equal opportunity clauses, love marriages that ended in divorce, beaten children who spent much of the day in the guidance office and away from class and a lot of alcohol-guzzling parents. What I saw, and no one spoke about, made me wonder why some people require eyeglasses and others do not.

In the fifth grade, a girl told me she would not sit next to me at lunch because I was handicapped: I thought it was my brown skin since that is what the British taught us Indians, but she explained that it was because I had four eyes. Her cruelty etched pain into my heart. I had become dependent after one year on eyeglasses and could not see without them any more. I began to wonder why people with eyeglasses are handicapped and what determined which eyes never got bent out of shape. In India, few people had eyeglasses. Was it that they were poor or that they had healthy eyes? Soon I was told bad vision was genetic and to stop asking questions.

Dr Jacob Liberman changed my view of eyesight during college. We had long discussions about the eyes and what he discovered from Australian aborigines. He explored the possibility of something impossible according to modern medicine: eyesight restoration without surgery. Through a series of exercises for the eyes and conditioning of the mind, which he has outlined in several of his books, he explains that we can modify our nervous system through heightened consciousness. The aborigines were yogis and knew how to transmute thoughts and the physical body.

Years later, an elderly wise man of Āyurveda talked to me about vision. Āyurveda tells us that the eyes adapt to aid the mind. If events in the environment are so perplexing for the mind that it cannot cope, the eyes also shift to seeing everything a little less clearly. Thus is the origin of myopia, the inability to see far away. Some yogis say that eye diseases are related to the inability of the mind to reconcile what it sees with what it believes to be real or right or good. The solution is to regularly yoke the mind with the emotions, the thoughts and exercises of the body so that everything stays connected and unclear thoughts are processed.

The Āyurvedic eye pharmacy that you can make at home for periodic cleansing as well as urgent needs will have rose water, ghee, honey, *mahatriphala ghrit, anjana*, a candle, a cucumber, heavy cream, maybe a mirror and will likely be located in the kitchen pantry. It will have nothing containing preservatives, remembering that the purpose of preservatives is to kill life in stagnant substances. Only rejuvenating substances, with clean hands, are put into the eye.

~ • 13 • ~

Cleaning the Senses: The Ears

Once a week, usually on a Sunday, my mother would lie all the little kids down in a row on a blanket. One by one, she would look in our ears—using a tug and pull—and occasionally, she would carefully use a bobby pin at the outer edge to scrape away anything that had accumulated. Then she would pour warm oil into our tiny ear canals and tell us to lie still as it soaked. It would put us to sleep. We learnt to never be afraid of ear examinations because the oil was so soothing. My father would coax us to participate, warning us that animals and bugs could be harboured in our ears and assuring us that oil would prevent monsters.

❧

Karnapurana is a time-tested, ancient ritual for re-establishing harmony in the ear. *Karna* is the Sanskrit word for ear, and *purana* means to fill. The practice suggests the filling of the ear canal with warm oil to moisten and seal the canal so that foreign organisms cannot penetrate, and loosen earwax.

The use of sesame oil has an anti-inflammatory and calming effect, as pure sesame oil reduces both *vāta* and *pitta*. The technique involves pouring warm, clean, pure sesame oil into the outer ear canal, letting it absorb for 15–20 minutes and then clearing the ear by sitting the patient up and facing the other side so that the oil drains directly out and not into the sinuses leading from the inner ear into the oral cavity. The oil must not be too warm, as it can burn, but it should not be cool as that is also irritating and certainly not comforting. Pouring is best done by soaking oil with gauze and gradually squeezing it near the opening of the ear canal so that the flow is smooth and droplets do not disturb the ear. A person will usually report an initial feeling of fullness and discomfort from decreased hearing and then enjoy the retreat from the outer senses.

A physician approached me warily after a *karnapurana* workshop with accusations of the unproven safeness and possible risk to the patient. I am always amused by these fearful professionals and 'experts' of the human body who never grew up living in and near human bodies enough to know common sense. Before starting, a parent will rub three fingers above the ear to ensure that the person can hear and that the eardrum is intact. An examination for pus or signs of pain precedes putting anything in the ear. If the ear has had no recent trauma, the child is not tugging the ear (indicating infection) or complaining of hearing changes or the child has had *karnapurana* since a young age, the practice is quite safe and is indeed quite effective at resolving many of the issues that require urgent medical interventions. The best way to learn these techniques is to watch, experience, participate and give.

A good Āyurvedic physician will tell you that *karnapurana* will pacify *vāta* and draw it out of the ear. The best way to understand this is to witness it. Once *karnapurana* is started, and the person is lying still, ear up towards the sky, oil filling the entire ear canal, a curious observer can watch the pool of oil. If the person has an excess of *vāta*, it manifests as movement out of the body. Bubbles start to emerge from the oil and continue to emerge. Āyurveda refers to this excess *vāta* in the head of the patient as disharmonized air that is slowly drawn out by filling the micropores of the body with oil. Recent neuroscience shows that pure oil will penetrate the brain through the nerve channels known as inter-axon canals, not through the blood and carry nutrients into the brain using pathways not recognized by mainstream medical science yet.

Steps for *karnapurana*:

- After ensuring there is no tear in the eardrum, have someone pour warm, clean pure sesame oil into the outer ear canal.
- Use gauze or cotton to soak the warm oil and gradually squeeze it near the opening of the ear canal so that it flows smoothly.
- Let it absorb for 15–20 minutes and then clear the ear by sitting up slowly, keeping the head directly forward and turning onto the opposite ear so that the oil drains directly out and not into the sinuses leading from the inner ear into the oral cavity.
- The oil must not be too warm or cool.

A busy industrialist living in Mumbai has an elderly nonagenarian mother that kept him tied to the city. He rarely travelled outside for more than a few days because his mother had a series of medical issues. Of course, they had access to the best doctors in the city and were able to get house calls from the city's finest.

One day, over tea at the Belvedere Club in the Oberoi, he confided that he was busy with yet another round of trips to neurologists in the city, trying to solve a decade-long problem that was again urgent. His mother had a balance problem and could never be left alone, as she would tip over or fall off her chair from intermittent dizziness. She could not stay in bed and had to be moved around to prevent sores from forming. Occasionally, she would get nauseated and vomit, so choking was a constant threat. Several full-time attendants would be in and out of their massive, wrap-around flat on Marine Drive each day.

His frustration and helplessness were obvious. I asked whether she had ringing in the ears, and he stared at me, affirming that she had been diagnosed with tinnitus by the best doctors, who had declared it incurable. Boldly, with my faith in the non-toxic nature of Āyurveda when properly applied, I asked if he wanted to try something. We went to his flat, and I demonstrated *karnapurana*, showing two attendants how to perform the same procedure and the precision of each step. After 20 minutes, she was fine. I prescribed warm sesame oil in the opposite ear for the next day, and if she was fine, I recommended sesame oil into each ear twice a day for 5 days. I suggested they then shift to *karnapurana* once a day for 2 weeks.

At the end of 5 days, the son called to tell me that his mother had woken up and called urgently for him. She had no ringing in her ears, and her mood had improved immediately. She had started eating more and had better bowel movements. He called 2 days later to let me know he had contacted the neurologist about the 'incurable' tinnitus, and the doctor had confessed that as a licensed modern medical doctor, he could not prescribe such simple cures, and that he had to prescribe what the medicine of his profession demanded. 'Never mind the patient', the industrialist scoffed. 'They worry more about their reputation than about healing their patients.'

Then he disappeared. After two months, he called again for advice. I asked why he had disappeared. 'Doctors are for the sick, not for the well,' he stated. After another week of treatment, his mother had improved steadily and all dizziness, nausea and balance issues had stopped. Suddenly, he had his mother back. So there was no time for anyone. His mother had one wish—to fly to the Golden Temple. So a chartered plane had rushed the mother, son and one caretaker to Amritsar, and they had enjoyed a balmy holiday walking together. Soon after coming back, some dizziness had restarted, and that is why he called.

As pleased as I was about the patient's recovery, I explained that *vāta* aggravation is common, and that the flight and travel had increased his mother's *vāta* again. Immediately, we started another round of daily *karnapurana*, and the symptoms again disappeared. A deeper course of food, lifestyle and Āyurvedic herbs for reducing *vāta* was discussed, along with a pharmacy in Mumbai where the driver could regularly buy the medicines. Years later, his mother continues to prosper.

The ear is the opening to a complex series of structures inside the head aligned to detect sound and interpreting it as hearing, for aiding the body to find balance and for orienting the body to gravity. Inside the flap—known as the pinna—is a long canal, at the end of which is the eardrum. The eardrum is very sensitive to vibrations and movements of air.

It is connected to the three bones of the ear behind the eardrum, in an area known as the middle ear. This is the site of most ear infections because a small thin canal connects this area to the back of the throat.

Beyond the three bones is the protected region of the inner ear. It is one of the most important areas of the body because it houses the semicircular canals and sensory organs that determine balance of the body in relation to gravity and detect motion around the body. It also contains the organ for hearing, known as the cochlea, with its snail-like shape.

Hearing is tested in a variety of ways, including sound tests and vibration on the bones of the skull. Many diseases slowly diminish a person's ability to hear and thus perceive stimuli in the environment. Āyurveda discusses toxins that build up in the ear, *vāta* that disturbs and eventually destroys the nervous system in the ear and the importance of emotions and the metaphor of sound, in which people stop hearing because they do not want to hear what they cannot take in.

The original language of the mind and its relationship to consciousness and the soul is said to be Sanskrit, which was preserved orally so that its profound effect could be transmitted through the ears to the brain. We start prayers, chants and rituals with the harmonic sound om, said to be the humming sound of Planet Earth zooming through space.

In the past three decades, Āyurveda has gradually ignored the resonance of Sanskrit, which espouses a philosophy of inherent connection with nature and its forces. Pressured by modern scientists and governmental/regulatory bodies to validate its principles using the language of biomedical science, the language of Sanskrit, as well as the culture around it known as *Sanskriti*, is losing its reflection as a science of understanding the universe in relation to consciousness.

Unlocking the deepest meanings in ancient Āyurvedic sūtras requires several languages, beyond Sanskrit and biomedical science. Several obstacles exist for translating Āyurveda from its original Sanskrit, the least of which is the grammar or construction. In fact, the grammar is similar to German and the construction is similar to computer languages. With its depth of intended multiple meanings for the same term and contextual references, the Sanskrit language emphasizes the understanding of subtle relationships.

In major universities of the world, it is widely held that Sanskrit is 'a dead language'. The news has not spread that there are over 7,00,000 Āyurvedic physicians, yogis and Sanskrit scholars who have a working knowledge of Sanskrit and use it regularly to consult their texts for clinical work.

This stems from the widespread tactic of spreading misinformation and affirming western supremacy. Reports such as 'The Education Reform Minute' of Macauley presented in 1833 in Calcutta (now Kolkata) led to the subjugation of Sanskrit in favour of English-medium education across all kingdoms of Bharat. The likely origin of Greek medicine from India was no longer conveyed. When India was formed, most of the laws regarding health and establishment of medical regulations were imported directly from British law books, heavily supporting the developing field of allopathic medicine and veering away from indigenous sciences as the backbone of the new country. These obstacles historically hindered sociopolitical awareness or a positive attitude towards Āyurveda and the importance of hearing Sanskrit. In addition, many Āyurvedic physicians today are not confident about their Sanskrit language skills, as students enrolling in Āyurvedic medical schools are no longer required to have formally studied a year of Sanskrit. It is said that understanding Sanskrit is understanding the science of life.

In the practice of family medicine, one of the most common complaints is ear infections in little kids or swimmers. After learning about the overuse of antibiotics and the statistic that most ear infections are viral and thus untreated by antibiotics, I started advising garlic oil. Known for its antibacterial and antiviral effects, its ability to penetrate the body with its volatile oils and its safety, I strongly advise parents to make fresh garlic oil and apply it to the first centimetre of the opening of their children's ears before allowing them to go swimming. A clove of garlic is peeled from its bulb and skin, then pounded on a non-porous surface, such as marble or ceramic, so that the oil is apparent. A swab is used to collect the oil from the surface and applied to the ear. During *karnapurana*, a clove of garlic can be warmed in a small pot of sesame oil, allowing some of the garlic oil to seep into the sesame oil base, which is then used to fill the ear that is prone to infection.

To treat ear infections, especially those caused by swimming in public pools, follow these steps:

- Separate a clove of garlic from the bulb and peel the skin.
- Pound it on a non-porous surface so that the fresh oil is apparent.
- Use a clean swab to collect it and apply it to the ear.
- For little children, parents can prepare fresh garlic oil and apply it to the first centimetre of the opening of their children's ears before swimming.

Even during *karnapurana*, a clove of garlic can be warmed along with the sesame oil so that garlic oil can seep into the sesame oil base. Use this to treat the affected ear.

❧

~ • 14 • ~

Cleaning the Senses: The Nose

Every so often, usually in the deep of winter, my mother would lay my father's head in her lap, as we all giggled and watched her apply oil to his face, then a moist, steamy washcloth. Then she would tilt his head far back and slowly squeeze two emerald droplets from a little white and brown bottle into his right nostril. He would inhale powerfully, snorting the drops deep into his head. She would repeat on the left nostril. Then she would rub his forehead and temples, and the region below his eyes for several minutes, massaging in the oil.

Suddenly, he would spring up from her lap, coughing, snorting and making sounds, and then run to the bathroom to drop a collection from his mouth. We would jump wildly, giggling and watching. My sister's favourite colour was green, and she was eager to experience the emerald medicine too, but my mother was adamant. It was not that it was only for boys, she said, but that the drops would go deep into the head and irritate little peoples' sinuses. So we learnt that the little bottle that sat on my father's grooming cabinet in the bathroom next to a little pot was not to be touched.

❧

The practice of *nasya* is considered one of the five great cleansings in Āyurveda, known as the *panchakarma*. *Nasya* is used to clean out mucous and toxins that have accumulated in the head and neck, gathering wastes from the crevices of the sinuses, nostrils, nasal cavity, mouth and throat.

While there are many options, *anu thailam* and *brahmi oil* are considered among the most common and most available formulations for the correct practice of *nasya*. A systematic process was developed 5000 years ago and elaborated upon by ancient scientists. Warming the head and neck, the blood flow was increased so that movement of contaminants stuck inside the body could be drawn out. Warm oil on the skin sealed the pores from leaking heat. A hot washcloth applied steam to heat the sinuses and hollow structures under the forehead, cheeks and face.

Tilting the head so that cleansing herbs in droplet form flowed down the nasal cavity would cause all the dirt and toxins to coalesce and draw them out. After they collected as the passages cooled naturally, the patient would sit up and use gravity to expel the collected phlegm from the entire connected network of passages leading outwards to the nose and mouth.

Regular *nasya* helps keep nasal passages clean for those who are healthy and gradually cleanses and cures the sinuses and hollows of those who are afflicted. It is used to heal a whole variety of diseases in the head as oil-based toxins are slowly drawn out over time. The sense of smell is rejuvenated, and nasal hairs, which protect against unwanted invasions of bacteria, grow healthy. In addition, open passages obviously increase the oxygen taken into the body.

❧

Placing things in the nose has recently been made illegal for anyone in the US except physicians, since it is considered a type of entrance into the body and thus a surgery. But the passages are continuous with the flow of air, so they are really open though convoluted. In fact, anyone guided properly can practise *nasya*.

There are many types of *nasya*, depending on the needs of the person, collected in ancient scripts over thousands of years of safe practice. An Āyurvedic physician will individualize recommendations to the person, depending on the environment, climate, season, lifestyle, workplace and logistics.

Sometimes, dry powders such as *brahmi* are used instead of oils, blowing them like snuff into the nose, like the first application of cowpox used in the 1700s by Jenner to vaccinate against smallpox in Europe. Called *pradhamana nasya*, powders are dry and thus mainly used to treat *kapha*-dominating diseases of heaviness, stickiness and stagnancy, such as headaches, common colds, heaviness in the head, nasal congestion, sticky collections of pus around the eyes and sinusitis. Advanced diseases of swelling of lymph nodes in the neck or skin immune diseases, nervousness, anxiety, fear, dizziness and emptiness are also treated by *pradhamana nasya* carefully by an experienced Āyurvedic physician. The powders penetrate and slowly dissolve into the fat-dominated immune system and slowly release their chemicals and *pitta*-pacifying elements into the plentiful immune cells in the head and neck. Neurological diseases, such as epilepsy, chronic drowsiness and parkinsonism are treated by *nasya* by competent Āyurvedic physicians for the same reason; nerve cells are bundled by fat and have their own transport system independent of the blood highways of the body.

Ghee *nasya* is a nutritive (*bruhana* in Sanskrit) *nasya*, loved by those who use ghee regularly. Since the head is oily and the passages are prone to phlegm, but also to dryness and roughness from the constant intake and outflow of air, ghee is a natural remedy for *vāta* and drying tendencies. *Bruhana nasya* uses *shatavari* ghee, *ashwagandha* ghee and medicated milk to cure dryness and *vāta* conditions in the head, along with oils, salts and plain ghee. Studies suggest it can improve *vāta*-type headaches, migraines, hoarse voice, dry nose and sinuses, loss of sense of smell, heavy eyelids, bursitis and stiffness in the neck, all consequences of excess dryness and roughness of the tissues. People also report less negative, dry thoughts that lead to nervousness, anxiety, fear, dizziness and emptiness as symbolically these are also *vāta* tendencies of the mind. Because Āyurveda does not distinguish between mind and body as much as modern medicine, all types of *vāta* conditions are cured using moist, warm and grounding oily formulations.

The lack of ability to sleep has become endemic in modern society. Ancients understood the cleansing power of good sleep and used *nasya* as a palliation or calming treatment to promote healthy, restful sleep. *Shamana nasya* is tailored to each person, noting whether imbalanced or excess *vāta*, *pitta*, or *kapha* is creating insomnia. Usually, agitation and *pitta* aggravation play a part, with inflammation in the head and neck. Hence, sedative *nasya* includes qualities opposite to *pitta*, using *pitta*-reducing and inflammation-reducing herbs as decoctions (known as *nāvana nasya*), teas and light oils. Ghees are too heavy and coagulate the heat of the inflammation. Liquids are more cooling by nature, invoking a smooth anti-*pitta* response. Within a couple of weeks, people report sound sleep, less snoring, less sleep apnoea and thus, often better night-time marital relations.

Kapha is the dominant *dosha* in the head and neck because of the high amount of fat and oil contained therein. In fact, 25 per cent of the body's cholesterol is used for brain membranes, which have to be super-smooth and super-fast to transmit our nerve impulses.

According to Āyurveda, *kapha* is the reflection of the qualities of earth and water, and it embodies the theme of stability and lubrication.

Earth and water are the heaviest of the five elements, and they are cool, stagnant, thick, cloudy and soft. The qualities of water are reflected both in *pitta* and *kapha*. The themes of stability and lubrication epitomize the brain and head, which oversee the vital functions. *Kapha*-dominating structures around the *vāta* functions counterbalance the cold, windy, dry flow—lubricating those passages so that the body maintains smoothness and supple strength.

Areas that are dominated by the principle of *kapha* include the lungs and structures around it in the chest that require smooth movement, the joint capsules containing synovial fluid and bursa fluid, the lining around the nerve cells and brain tissues, and the upper portion of the digestive system (in the mouth and upper stomach).

Excess lubrication that becomes sticky and builds up is abnormal *kapha*. Diseases in which lubrication or stability are imbalanced are *kapha* diseases. When the head is filled with phlegm and mucous, too much moisture and too much stickiness, the area is *kapha*-imbalanced. As the heaviness builds up and prevents normal flow and function, *kapha* aggravation occurs. The result is decreased strength of the tissues. The heat of normal fire in the body keeps *kapha* in check. Movement by *vāta* moves the heaviness of *kapha* along in the body. Āyurveda interpreted the signs and symptoms as a whole with the term *kapha*.

❧

The main function of the nose organ is to smell. It also acts to warm the air breathed in before it travels inward to the depth of the chest and lungs, where excess cool air can cause constriction. The nose also humidifies dry air to reduce excess dryness from entering the lungs. The hairs in the nose remove unwanted particles from the air, preventing unnecessary contamination and infections of the lungs.

As air passes over the specialized cells lining the nose in the olfactory epithelium which lines the sinuses behind the nose and eyes, the receptors detect these airborne chemicals, sending signals to the brain, which then identifies known and foreign smells. Humans have about 350 different types of smell receptors, which connect via nerve cells to the olfactory bulb located in the oldest part of the brain, the paleoencephalon. From there, the signals go to a myriad of locations in the brain associated with both emotional and physiological responses to the odour. This is why odours, even after a long lapse of smelling a particular fragrance, will revive old visual, auditory and location memories.

My best friend from college eventually became an anaesthesiologist. Over the years of his training, I watched his nose turn chronically red and his eyes itch and water at each change of weather, any smoke or pollution, pollen or excess heat. After a decade of chronic sinusitis, unable to breathe or speak smoothly, he finally revealed his addiction to nose drops every half hour, and the ineffectiveness of every possible anti-histamine and sinusitis medicine, including experimental therapies. He had become unable to teach a full hour of class, and he was sleep-deprived. It never occurred to him that breathing anaesthesia gases in the operating room over a decade of work, 15 hours a day, had any association with his chronic sinusitis.

Finally, exasperated, he asked me about 'that ancient Āyurveda stuff'. It is common for people to wait until allopathic drugs fail, rather than consider the source of an imbalance before it becomes a chronic illness. In the beginning, I decided to just help him breathe as quickly as possible, saving underlying curative treatments for later, if he decided to continue with Āyurveda. Called *srotosodhana*, I showed him how to slowly inhale warm water into one nostril, holding the other nostril closed.

After a moment, a strong exhale would expel all the water, as well as any loose phlegm or mucous that was in the nostril. After two inhales on the right side, I instructed him to repeat the procedure on the left. Of course, one nostril was always full and he was unable to do a full inhale and exhale completely in the beginning. But after 2 days he reported that he could draw water in from both sides. That made him more curious, as he recalled, 'I knew I could take water into my nose, because I did it when I went swimming. But it went straight into my head and irritated me, so I always thought it was dangerous.' Once he analysed what he was doing, in a controlled way, he allayed his fears.

We proceeded with *jalneti* and a *neti* pot. *Jal* means water in Sanskrit, and *neti* means to wash.

He laughed at the genie bottle, a smooth elegant oblong pot like a kettle with a spout on one end, hole pointed upward. I instructed him to take a quart of tepid water and add one teaspoon of sea salt and a quarter teaspoon of turmeric powder. After stirring, the head needed to be tilted sideways downward. I showed him by placing my finger along the side of my nose, and bending until the third knuckle at the base of the finger was higher than the fingernail. This meant the head was low enough for water to flow properly.

In this position, the spout of the *neti* pot was to be firmly inserted into the nostril and the water from the pot was to be slowly poured into the nostril. Eventually, it would flow out of the other nostril. My friend considered the proposition carefully. Of course he had lots of questions. Did the water have to be distilled or sterile? What temperature is tepid? What happened if the turmeric stained his towel or the sink? What if the water just did not come out the other side and went into the head? What if his vision got blurry? What if he vomited? How precise did the measurements of salt and turmeric have to be?

After all the questions were settled, he leaned over, holding his finger along the slant of his nose, placing the fingernail near the tear gland of his eye, glancing tentatively at me. We inserted the spout and began to pour the warm water. To his concern and amazement, after about 10 seconds, water began to flow out of his left nostril and into the basin. After the pot was empty, it was refilled with a second dose of warm salted turmeric water and firmly inserted into the left nostril, and water happily flowed out of the right nostril.

This process was to be done twice a day, in the morning on waking and in the evening before bed, or at least after coming home from a chemical-filled day of work. After a week of adjusting to the routine, I suggested he increase the turmeric, due to its natural antibiotic and anti-inflammatory properties, to half a teaspoon of turmeric powder in each quart. After 3 weeks, I suggested he put a drop of mustard oil on his finger and coat the inside of his nostrils before bed, to coat and soothe.

After several weeks of feeling better, a voice from the past telephoned; it was my friend from college, with no nasal stuffy voice or sniffling. He revealed his anger at our own profession of allopathy, which does not teach physicians how to care for bodies in different ways. He asked me to unravel how I approached severe and chronic sinusitis and how to guide his students and colleagues who seemed to have similar trajectories of illness.

For anyone who opens their mind to what they have observed in the world, Āyurvedic *dosha*s are obvious. The three *dosha*s in the body get muddled from all the foreign toxins and unnatural lifestyle in a typical hospital environment, creating sinusitis. In medical terms, dry air in the operating room dries the nostrils over time, creating micro-cracks in the mucous layer inside the nose.

Airborne toxins from chemicals, patients and cleansers in operating rooms find their way into the microscopic cracks and wedge in, creating a warning for the body, which sends in immune system soldiers to attack the foreign particles. These immune cells release their defences, including histamine to call in more soldiers, killing bacteria but also human cells, and they release fluids as they flood the nostrils to do their work. The result is a runny nose, itching from the histamine, redness from all the inflammatory chemicals of the immune system and a stuffy nose from all the fluids.

In Āyurvedic terms, since sinusitis is an inflammation as well as a chronic build-up of mucous, it is a *pitta–kapha* disturbance. Āyurveda did not use cells and the biochemical language of immunology. It talks of patterns of the forces of nature: toxins lodge in the nose, things that feel unnatural because they are drying, cold, rough and thus irritating. The body reacts to this irritation by producing heat, sharpness and increasing blood flow to the area, increasing *pitta*. The congestion and reactive production of mucous, known as *kleda*, to counter the dryness and roughness, creates a snuffy nose, excess phlegm and runny nose, and *kapha* aggravation.

The solution in Āyurveda is to reduce *pitta* and *kapha* through a balance of herbs and substances that are compatible with the tissues inside the nose and mouth. *Jalneti* is considered a clean and easy wash that can access the sinuses gradually and regularly, coating the nostrils with water so that cracks can heal. Mustard oil coats, soothes and reduces *kapha*. Turmeric balances all the *dosha*s, and salt breaks down the *kapha–kleda* phlegm. Oil drops at night, especially in the dry winter, and a regular practice of *jalneti* to balance the life choice of working in the operating rooms or any dry environment, helps maintain the balance of the body.

❧

Daily lubrication for the nose is formally known in Āyurveda as *pratimarshya nasya.* It is quick and easy, and is often the only recommendation many of my busy, non-meditative patients will follow. Usually done at night so that the nostril does not point downward, *pratimarshya nasya* can be done on a regular basis and while travelling. The clean little finger is dipped in a small bottle of ghee or oil kept separately for the purpose and inserted into each nostril. After inserting the finger, the nasal passage becomes lubricated. From the outside, the nostril is gently massaged to open the deep nasal tissues.

~ • 15 • ~

Cleaning the Senses: The Skin

As a tween, I began spending more time out in the world without my mother. The consumption of French fries and chocolate, and time in the hot sun along with the onset of adolescence began to reflect on my darkened face as whiteheads, pus-filled mountains or black-topped hills. I would awaken and spend time lamenting in front of the mirror, unable to make the connection between my habits and what was attacking my face. Babi and my elder sister still had scars of their lost war with acne, and I looked at my mother, as radiant as ever, with a smooth complexion and no wrinkles.

She showed me her stick of sandalwood, demonstrating how to grind the hardwood on the grinding flat stone she had used for decades, to bring out a white–beige paste that she would spread across her face. She discussed how precious the wood is and therefore, asked me to use the wood only if I would commit to doing it each and every night. I took on the challenge to improve myself, a kind of *sadhana*, and applied the paste to my washed face each and every night before bed. In the morning, my face was tighter and over time it became shades lighter, soft and devoid of all blemishes and craters. After a month of commitment and success, my mother presented me with my own stick and grinding stone. The routine continued into my twenties, and then occasionally for a few weeks at a time when stress-induced outbreaks occurred. That same stick and stone is with me now, more valuable than ever, since white sandalwood is now endangered and highly regulated by trade. The authentic wood with its fragrant oils must be grown in the proper soil, is rarely available and thus one of the most expensive woods.

Increasing data on the benefits of basking in the rays of the rising sun counterbalance the data on melanomas and the need for sunscreen and protection from the sun. The Sanskrit sloka from the Matsya Purana, one of the ancient books of Indian philosophy, tells us that *arogyam bhaskara-dichhet* (early morning sun rays) are the giver of good health.

Considered the oldest systematic philosophy and science conceived by man and continuously followed through time to the present day, the Vedas are not a religion but rather a world view of living in alignment with the subtle forces of nature. Written circa 10,000 years BCE, the Vedas describe forces only recently discovered by physics and chemistry. Several rituals emphasized the importance of the early rising sun, including Surya Namaskar, a series of yoga movements facing the morning sun, with mantras to be evoked facing it, like the one my mother does each morning.

Of course, biology tells us that the biosphere is sustained by the sun, and weather patterns are deeply affected by the undulating heating and cooling during rotation and revolution of the earth around the sun. But there was something specific about the rays of the morning sun being more beneficial than its rays at any other time of day. The ninth chapter of the Atharva Veda describes twenty-two diseases that can be cured by the rays of the rising sun.

The Vedas claim that the sun can heal heart problems, jaundice and anaemia. Long ridiculed as far-fetched claims, science is now discovering the importance of vitamin D, produced by the skin from the sun, in modulating hormones and enzymes that affect the heart and blood. Indeed, premature babies are laid in incubators with UV light to cure their neonatal jaundice. Over a thousand different genes, governing almost every tissue in the body, are now known to be regulated by the active form of the vitamin D_3, including several involved in calcium metabolism, endorphin and pain regulation, blood pressure through modulation of renin in the kidneys and the optimal functioning of the neuromuscular and immune systems. There is also a connection between vitamin D deficiency and the development of diabetes and the metabolic syndrome. Vitamin D also induces cathelicidin, a polypeptide that effectively combats both bacterial and viral infections.

When people are exposed to sunlight or very bright artificial light in the morning, their nocturnal melatonin production occurs sooner, and they enter into sleep more easily at night. This hormone from the pineal gland also plays an important role in countering infection, inflammation, cancer and auto-immunity.

Unprotected sunlight exposure has been discouraged mainly due to melanoma risk. However, reports also state that 0.1 per cent of the human population is at risk of UV-light-related diseases, whereas 50 per cent of the human population is at risk of other diseases from lack of sunlight exposure. The safest compromise seems to be to take in sunlight when the UV Index is low. In general, the intensity of UV rays at the end of the day is higher than at the beginning of the day.

~ • 16 • ~

Cleaning the Senses: The Mouth

Every morning as a child, without fail, I would hear a series of gargling emanating from windows around the neighbourhood in Santoshpur. They would vary in depth, duration and tone. But they were a signal that people had woken and were cleaning themselves for a new day. After we moved to Princeton, my father continued his routine with the same fervour, gargling loudly and strongly for as long as he could hold the liquid in his mouth.

A neighbour, dignified and repressed about bodily functions and the noises they emanate, came politely to our apartment one day to tell my mother that this was not how things were done in the civilized society of America. People should not reveal noises from their bodies through any opening. My mother listened politely, offered another cup of tea and cake and using her best European manners, bid the visitor goodbye. She then struggled to find a way to tell my father that the neighbours did not want to hear him gargle. Over the next several weeks, my parents tried several things; they closed the windows in the bathroom and adjoining bedrooms; they opened the water faucets so that it was very loud. Finally, my father installed a loudspeaker radio and turned the channel to morning news, turning the volume up for the 2 minutes that he gargled. My parents gargled at the same time to economize. After they turned down the volume, my little ears wondered why, curiously, they could hear other noises emanating from spastic bellies and cigarette coughs, spouses yelling at their spouses and families, and various eruptions from the bodies of these civilized people.

Mouthwash has been popularized by professional dentists in the last fifty years as a method for getting to the crevices of the teeth and mouth where toothbrush and foamy toothpaste do not succeed, mainly for cleaning plaque from teeth and freshening the mouth. The thin liquids contain sweeteners, alcohol and detergents, as well as chemicals to leave a cool taste in the mouth.

mukhavairasyadaurgandhyaśōphajāḍyaharaṁ sukham |
danta-dārḍhyakaraṁ rucyaṁ snēha-gaṇḍūṣa-dhāraṇam ||14||

Gargling with oil removes bad taste, bad smells, inflammation and feelings of numbness in the mouth and is pleasant, strengthens the teeth and promotes the natural affinity for food. |

Suśruta Samhita,
Cikitsa-sthāna; chapter 24, sloka 14

During medical school, one of my friends began to clench his teeth. He complained regularly of pain in his left jaw under his ear. He could no longer chew gum, bite down on hard objects or open his mouth wide to sing. The pain was so severe that sometimes he would sit in class and massage his cheeks or behind his ear. Eventually, after a clicking noise appeared when he opened his mouth, he went to the dentist and was told his back teeth were wearing down and in danger of eventual replacement.

Diagnosed as temporal mandibular junction (TMJ) disorder, he was told that he was in danger of damaging his tongue as he grinded his teeth and clenched his jaw unconsciously in his sleep. A teeth guard was made for his mouth, and he was instructed to wear this every night. Sheepishly, he asked how long he would have to wear it and was told that it should be used until he eventually stopped grinding, which could be for life. There was no cure for TMJ disorders.

The TMJ is the joint between the front lower edge of the skull, just under the ears and the large crescent-shaped jawbone that holds the lower teeth and shapes the jawline. There are two TMJs, one on each side of the jaw. The joint is designed for up-and-down movement, with some small flexibility for other angles, and allows for chewing, biting and talking.

Modern medicine estimates there are millions of people with TMJ disorders and has spent years and money in research to understand the causes and potential treatments of these. Surgery, implants, botulinum toxin A and bite guards have been researched, as well as acupuncture, osteopathic treatments, chiropractic and massage therapy.

Since the time of Āyurveda, wise men advised about the importance of daily swishing before and after brushing, to condition both the inside and outside muscles of the mouth. For more serious problems, they advised the invested ritual of the mouth, *gandusha*.

Gandusha is the systematic holding of medicated oils in the mouth to cure chronic problems as well as strengthen the oral cavity's normal functions. Analysing the composition and functions of the mouth, Āyurveda doctors composed a recipe and delivery form that fortifies the unctuousness of the surfaces, the strength of the teeth and the suppleness of the muscles.

One of my medical students came to me after her dental visit, describing her new diagnosis of TMJ disorder. Explaining that she had started grinding her teeth and clicking at night, according to her boyfriend, she had noticed increasing pain in her right jaw since the second year of medical school. She also noticed that she clenched her jaw during exams. Interested in holistic treatments, she wanted to find a natural solution, rather than investing in a bite guard, which the dentist was only too happy to make for her and which was not curative. She wanted to address the root of the problem.

The simplest way of doing *gandusha*, known as oil pulling in the west, is to use sesame oil. In the first phase, she swished with warm water for half a minute, then applied a thick coat of warm sesame oil to the inside of her mouth, tracing from the back recesses of the inner cheek pouch out toward the lips. Then she filled her mouth with warm water and held it until her eyes and nose watered, usually 2–3 minutes. Then she was to pour out the water from her mouth into the bathroom sink and look for the colour. She was to do this twice a day for 2 weeks, and then report to me for phase two.

Oil applied to the inside cheeks seeps its way through the mucous lining into the channels that line the nerve cells. It remoistens them and promotes proper nerve flow, reducing pain. According to Āyurveda, pain in the joints is a *vāta* disorder, caused by microscopic dryness, roughness and lack of proper movement along the body's micro-channels. It also stimulates parotid glands and lymph nodes, which are plentiful in the oral cavity.

2 weeks later, a twinkling student returned to me, eager to begin phase two. She reported noticeable relief within days of

starting, though she admitted that it was initially difficult to control gagging reflexes while holding water in the mouth after lining the mouth with oil. While she was reportedly still grinding her teeth at night, she was experiencing a lot less pain. The yellow oil turned white when she spit it out, and she wondered why. I explained to her that sesame oil pulls out toxins which turn the oil white. It lowers *vāta*, and quickly and strongly allays pain, microscopic dryness and roughness. The swishing, known in Sanskrit as *kavala*, pulls out toxins, while the retention during *gandusha* penetrates and lubricates.

For phase two, now that she had mentally accepted the idea of heavy oil in her mouth, she began swishing then gargling with the sesame oil, filling the mouth and swishing for 2 minutes, then taking a deep breath and gargling for as long as she could, allowing the oil to penetrate into the lower throat and glands. When she spit out the contents from her mouth, again she was to notice the colour.

After another month, she returned to report that she was no longer grinding. Her boyfriend was joyous that she was again silent in her sleep, and she did not clench her jaw during the recent round of exams that she had endured. To ensure that the clenching did not return, she started a small daily yoga routine of face yoga and Surya Namaskar, with some stretching both on waking and before bed. I also encouraged her to spend more emotional time with her boyfriend and loved ones, and to unwind daily so that the pressures of medical school did not implode in her closed mouth.

According to Āyurveda, the practice of *gandusha* strengthens the teeth when done regularly. It enhances the strength of the mandible and the resonance of the voice, nourishes and lubricates the facial nerves, improves taste sensation and promotes better function of the taste buds by pulling oil-soluble toxins and imbalanced *dosha*s from the mouth. As needed, herb decoctions can be boiled into the oil by knowledgeable Āyurvedic physicians to make medicated oil, using turmeric, honey, *triphala* and *khadira*. With regular use, *gandusha* prevents dryness of the throat, cracking of the lips and decay of the teeth because it adds moisture and smoothness through oil into the microscopic layers of the mouth.

Āyurveda also advises that too much of a good thing is not therapeutic. Too much *gandusha* can lead to mouth ulceration, diseases in the mouth from excess *kapha* and excessive thirst with loss of taste due to over-coating of the taste buds. Therefore, once a week in the oily months of summer, and twice a week in the dry and cold months is a good maintenance plan for those who want to use *gandusha* as a *rasayana* (rejuvenating treatment).

In ancient Āyurveda texts, the last section describing the care of the mouth advises *tambula*—the chewing of medicated betel leaves and holding fragrant substances in the mouth. Upon waking, after meals, before and after sex, and after vomiting, slightly scented, pungent and/or astringent herbs are spread on betel leaves, which are neatly folded and inserted into the pocket of the mouth and chewed slowly. *Tambula*, or paan, slowly cleanses, eliminates bad breath and tones the voice. Usual substances for preparing *paan* include *supari* (betel nut), clove, nutmeg, black pepper, limes and catechu. *Tambula* is enjoyed as a festive delicacy but has increasingly become an addiction in Indians over the centuries as the combination of sweet and astringent is alluring and provides a boost of energy. *Paan* sellers abound lucratively on the streets of any town where Indians live.

The alternative is the use of fragrant herbs without betel leaves. Since childhood, all of my father's fine suits hid 2–3 cloves or cardamom pods in one of the pockets. As I began to secretly wear his older jackets that he rarely used, I found myself chewing on these and replenishing them from my mother's stock in her kitchens.

By adulthood, all of my handbags and backpacks held a few cloves, cinnamon bark or cardamom pods. During medical school and residency, the dress code forbade the chewing of gum, deeming it unprofessional. After fifty-hour shifts of non-stop, gruelling work however, my breath was more unprofessional, especially as I needed to approach patients, their family members, nurses and technicians regularly. I began to suck on cloves or cardamom seeds, which were easily hidden and discreet.

Āyurveda advises the use of sweet and sensual things coming into the being and the power of ingestion to inspire our thoughts. Use of these herbs also allows us to start the day by radiating fragrance from the body and from the mouth.

❧

The Voice

As soon as my father was safely out of the driveway, my mother would begin singing, starting with the scales and working into three-note sequences. Slowly, we learnt to follow and find our '*sa*'. It was not that my father did not like music, but the sound of my mother's perfect voice, recruited for All India Radio with its range and volume, reminded him of what he did not let her have and of the silence that she chose in the times she could have been vociferous.

She would take us through *sa re ga ma pa dha ni* to *ša*, and if all our little voices were inclined, the harmonium would emerge from its mahogany box, and my mother would guide us along in one of her favourite Rabindrasangeet. She taught us not to sing from our vocal cords or diaphragm, as we were learning from our choir teacher. She would point below our umbilicus, indicating that the voice comes from the deepest within, the *nabhi* and the second chakra, and moves up through a secret channel to the heart, up to the throat and out finally through the mouth.

Music is often considered a language, with coded meanings in each frequency of sound. Sound travels in waves, and waves that oscillate through the air in coordinated patterns create harmonic sound. Ancient shastras, texts of knowledge conceived by man, had three sciences related to the therapeutic use of sound. The deepest meanings of Sanskrit and the etiology of its terms requires entry into the esoteric realms of its connection with the science of sound and sound energy, which arose from Vedic understandings of vibrations, energy–matter relationships and the yoga of the mind. The ancient Indian system of *Nāda* yoga studied the effects of sound intonations on the human body, prescribing specific sounds to manifest particular effects in the mind. It is said that the Sanskrit phonemes/*shabda* themselves reveal the nature of reality.

The Gandharva Veda has been popularized in the past century, referring to an appendix of the Sama Veda containing 36,000 slokas, which outlined the basis for the Bharata Natya Shastra, one of the oldest texts of music science. Some suggest that *Bharata* is an acronym for the three syllables: *bha* for *bhāva* (mood), *rā* for rāga (melodic framework) and *ta* for *tāla* (rhythm), emphasizing the importance of sound and music in the subcontinent. The Gandharva Veda correlates it with the vibrations that integrate consciousness with the cycles and rhythms in our physiology, including the heart rhythms, our daily waking–sleeping circadian rhythm and our cyclic hormonal rhythms of our adrenalin, cortisol and melatonin.

Nāda yoga is the use of sound waves to affect the yoking of the conscious mind to the soul and deep meditation. *Nāda* means sound vibration. This philosophical approach to healing sees all physical matter and particles as energy in very slow motion. If sound energy actually forms the building blocks of the cosmos, then each physical entity is linked to a denser manifestation of a sound. *Nāda* yoga uses sound vibrations and resonances that correlate to the body to work on balancing the mind. It emphasizes the power of internal music, called *anahata*, to flow through subtle energy levels. Yogis practise deep inner vigilance to access the silence from which subtle vibrations give out messages.

Rāga *chikitsa* is the therapeutic use of patterns of music in structured melodies to affect the body's physiology. The rāgas of Indian classical music are used at prescribed *prahāras* to send medicinal vibrations through musical tones into the body and the nervous system. The elders of Indian classical music—such as Tansen—and descendants of musical geniuses—such as Baba Allaudin Khan—learnt rāgas for their effects on the human condition and reflexively played certain rāgas for certain moods or for particular health. For example, his son Ali Akbar Khan played Rāga Marwa to alleviate the distress of grieving and Rāga Sohni for headaches. Rāga Bageshri was played for insomnia, Rāga Deepak for gastic hyperacidity and Rāga Bhairavi in the early morning hours for high blood pressure. As a child, my father would play Ustad Bismillah Khan and his shehnai in the late evening, broadcasting Rāga Shivaranjani through the house as we finished our homework. It was used to improve intelligence.

Physicians will scoff at the unscientific nature of these Vedic applications of music claiming to healing the body. A regular use of classical Indian music however, will not cause side effects, gouge the wallet or create drug–drug interactions. And, if one day, the physics of sound catches up to the Vedic understanding of music and consciousness, scientists may find in their language that these sounds do create changes in the brain or hormone levels or neurotransmitters linking them with health conditions.

One of the only languages that integrated anatomy of the oral cavity with linguistics is Sanskrit. Lessons in Sanskrit often begin with the stretching of the mouth muscles by hyper-pronouncing the ten plus five vowels. The alphabet is then arranged in the order of sound emerging from positioning at the back of the mouth moving forward to positioning at the lips.

My mother would sit with the bright pink books—called *pratham bhag*, *ditiya bhag* and *tritiya bhag*—and a wooden spoon. With the spoon, she would mark exactly timed beats, called *laya*, and occasionally slap our palms if we lost focus or did not repeat after her properly. She would begin with the sounds emerging from the back of the tongue. Called guttural sounds, they are formed by squeezing the vocal cords and curling the tongue into a curve to make the sounds *k* and *g*. Aspirated with some force from the vocal cords, these sounds become *kh* and *gh*. These four form the first line of the Sanskrit alphabet.

Each subsequent line of the varnamala or Sanskrit alphabet was formed from sounds emerging from spots gradually further forward in the mouth. The second line uses the palatal region to make the sounds ch and jh. The third line is known as the cerebral or retroflex position. The dental position creates the sounds of the fourth line of the Sanskrit alphabet. The fifth line formed from the sounds of the tip of the tongue touching the lips lightly to make the sounds p and b is of labial sounds. Aspirated with some force from the vocal cords, these sounds become ph and bh. Along the right end of the first five lines are the corresponding nasals ong, ñ, n., n, and m. In addition, there are three s sounds, called sibilants, a palatal, a retroflex and lower dental. Then there are four semi-vowels, y, r, l, v and one aspirated empty sound, h.

The fourteen vowels were the toughest. Regional variations in the way vowels are released create differences in accents, interpretations and subtle meanings. Originally, my mother showed us the Bengali way for everyday use and then altered each to the Sanskrit pronunciation, which had an inexplicable resonance.

It is said that meditative powers are invoked when Sanskrit is pronounced correctly. But what do we do about regional variants, accents and other diversities in the expression of a language? Sanskrit tried to preserve the oral accuracy of sound by grounding it in the physical world from where the sounds were generated. When pronounced correctly, these letters give full exercise to the tongue and allow the mind to hear nuances of sound that are often not heard by monolingual speakers.

❧

During my months on call in paediatrics during medical residency, I had to work with very sick children. Some had low mental function due to their illnesses, the side effects of medications they were given, or from the chemotherapy that left them bald, tired and in a stupor.

My job, assigned by the sadist residents and attending physicians, demanded drawing blood from the children daily, as though micromanaging their numbers would heal them. I also had to manage to measure vital signs and information about their physical condition by poking and prodding. One day, as I tried to soothe myself from the painful work of pushing needles into little arms, hands and legs, I began to sing around the children. Hearing a voice with a joyous song, the children responded, smiling and watching intently as song erupted into their usually silent and monotonous lives.

Over the month, I began to bring music into the room, not the rock-n-roll of popular America, but a classical Indian voice, instrumental music, soothing tunes of drone music, new-age music and pieces used in music therapy. I sang songs I had learnt in my childhood. The children would become calmer, released from discomfort for a few moments.

As years pass, the evidence for music therapy in the medical setting accumulates. What is the reason that the sound of the voice is delightful? Āyurveda tells us that the voice is the most precise instrument of music, and that the voice has the capability of connecting us with the divine.

❧

To keep the voice healthy, medicated herbs needed to be introduced into the throat periodically. Lozenges, teas and gargling work, but they touch deep into the throat for just moments. Āyurveda spent considerable time developing delivery forms for its medicines, addressing the concerns of ease of use, pleasant taste, stability in final form, ease of transport, schedule for consumption, delivery to the site in the body needed and adherence by the patient.

To deliver herbs to the deep throat, the wise men of Āyurveda sought a form that would deliver particles to a highway of constant movement of air from birth until death, where fingers do not easily reach. They watched nature and how nature delivered things from one place to another.

It is not difficult to suppose that a wise man found someone coughing after inhaling ashes and smoke from a cooking fire. From this, the pharmaceutical delivery of medicines via *dhoompana* was born. Medicinal smoking is not new to man. Many cultures ritually smoke plants, lighting leaves, herbs and powders on fire, to inhale the smoke. *Dhoompana* is a systematic prescription of particular elements that will moisturize and clean the throat and vocal cords, remove dryness, and roughness, and replace phlegm with clean mucous provoked from the throat's rejuvenating mechanisms. The ancient shastras say that vitiated *kapha* in the head is eliminated most quickly by *dhoompana*, the drinking of smoke.

There are many varieties of *dhoompana*: for soothing coughs, for drawing up and out toxins, for moisturizing the dry throat and for eliminating waste. A typical routine in Āyurveda is the smoking of a clove in *dhoompana* in the winter months to soothe a sore throat and melt mucous.

The method for medicinal smoking is also precise. Smoke is first drawn in through the nose and then the mouth, but it is always exhaled through the mouth, as the toxins should never come through the nose, where it can travel to the space near the eyes. One should always smear some ghee or oil on the end and ignite it, so that the *dhoompana* is not completely dry and full of ash, and one should use an instrument to hold the herb. Sometimes, the smoke is drawn through a water vessel, called a *hookah*, so that the smoke is moistened. At times, the herbs are crushed and made into herbal cigarettes for ease of transport and storage.

The best times for *dhoompana* are just after bathing, eating, scraping the tongue, after brushing the teeth, after sneezing and after applying oils to the face (for example, after *nasya* or collyrium) and just after sleep. Common herbs include *kanchnar guggul*, a great scraping (*lekhaniya*) herb for all things *kapha*, especially in the neck and throat, which I use at the end of a common cold, for thyroid conditions, enlarged lymph nodes in the neck and throat, as well as in the case of formations of tumours in the neck and throat. Licorice (*yashtimadhu*) is a demulcent for those thick mucous coughs at the end of a bout of bronchitis or a bad cold. It can be smoked or added to teas and decoctions. Herbs such as cloves and cardamom also soothe the voice.

Āyurveda mentions a host of diseases and conditions in the face, head and neck that show great results with *dhoompana*. It prevents strong *vāta–kapha* disorders that occur above the shoulders. But it must be done with care at the correct times in the day's routine, and not in excess, in order to deliver the *dosha*-balancing agents according to the *vāta–pitta–kapha* flows of the day and the body. *Dhoompana* is not the same as a casual smoke of a cigarette; it is a planned medicinal application of smoke to the throat using the principles of Āyurvedic *dosha* and *guna* theories to balance the imbalances. If done improperly, without the guidance of someone that can diagnose *dosha*s and *guna*s, *dhoompana* can cause bleeding disorders, malfunctioning of the senses and mental disorientation. But if done well, at the right time, *dhoompana* liquefies the *kapha* in the chest, throat and head in minutes without drying, creating thirst or changes in function.

If done properly, *dhoompana* can be used to soothe coughs, draw up and out toxins, moisturize the dry throat and eliminate waste. But it must be done with care at the correct times in the day's routine, and not in excess. If done improperly, without the guidance of someone that can diagnose *dosha*s and *guna*s, *dhoompana* can cause bleeding disorders, malfunctioning of the senses and mental disorientation.

To prepare the *dhoompana*,

- Smear some ghee or oil on the end before igniting the herb.
- Use an instrument to hold it.
- A water vessel (hookah) may be used, and some herbs may be rolled into herbal cigarettes.

To smoke the *dhoompana*,

- First draw in smoke through the nose and then the mouth, but always exhale through the mouth.

The best times for *dhoompana* are just after bathing, eating, scraping the tongue, after brushing the teeth, after sneezing and after applying oils to the face and just after sleep.

- *Kanchnar guggul* is great for common cold, thyroid conditions, enlarged lymph nodes in the neck and throat, as well as some tumours in the neck and throat.
- Licorice (*yashtimadhu*) is effective against thick mucous coughs at the end of a bout of bronchitis or a bad cold. It can be smoked or added to teas and decoctions.
- Herbs such as cloves and cardamom soothe the voice.

Cleaning the Senses: Practical

The start of the day differs from person to person, depending on their routine, family, the season and the location. Āyurveda acknowledged these individual variations and advised the only constant—rebalancing the *dosha*s and *guna*s wherever they had become imbalanced. The rituals for cleaning the eyes, ears, nose, throat and mouth were not to be used every day throughout life; they were options depending on the imbalances the environment created. Rejuvenation routines often make use of these rituals as part of *rasayana* regimens, remembering the principle that the body is *sheeta*, *snigdha* and *agneya*, and requires those *guna*s to be replenished regularly in order to support healthy themes of movement, transformation, lubrication and stability in the body.

Because no definitive prescription can be outlined for every person, Āyurveda is often discarded as unscientific. Its proper use, however, allows any individual to savour rituals as they realign, rejuvenate and re-inspire a person to take control of the body, mind, senses and soul.

The best way to incorporate the rituals is to become familiar with them as they are needed, then create a mental checklist, running through the senses each day when completing the early morning routine. Any areas that call for attention require a planned course for a few days, a week or a month.

An Āyurvedic home pharmacy that promotes easy periodic cleansing, as well as facilitates urgent needs, is usually located near the kitchen and should include items for the eyes, such as rose water, ghee, honey, *mahatriphala ghrit*, *anjana*, a candle, a cucumber, heavy cream and maybe a mirror. None of the substances should contain preservatives, as their purpose is to kill life. Only rejuvenating substances, with clean hands, are put into the eye. For the ears, keep a small glass bottle of sesame oil, some cotton gauze, a small bowl, some ear buds and a garlic press. For the nose, procure a *neti* pot, a small jar of turmeric powder, some sea salt and cloves for *dhoompana*. For the throat and mouth, keep sealed glass jars of licorice and *kanchnār guggul*, cardamom, cloves and cinnamon. As you build the pharmacy, you will add your own personal notes and make it your own, to balance the *dosha*s in the ways they tend to imbalance in your own life and lifestyle.

Part III:
The Bath

After the morning cup of tea, watching the sunrise and sharing brief words, my now elderly father asks for today's agenda. Sensing my mother is awake, he begins his journey upstairs to start his daily bath routine. Even after the stroke has paralysed his right half, he cannot accept the beginning of a day without the rituals of his bath.

When we were younger, we could assist with the preparatory processes, but now as we have matured into womanhood, Babi quietly rises alone and heads toward his bathroom. He takes an hour or two to complete the entire process meditatively, using his one hand to balance himself in and out of the tub. We listen carefully from outside while he goes through his routine for any signs of distress. Else, we know he will emerge daily, as he has for decades. Though it is a big risk to let him bathe alone, we know that this ritual is one of his only ways of proving to himself that he is still his own person, responsible for his own body.

❧

Āyurveda does not specify one particular time of day for the bath, but it specifies a checklist and order for tasks. The optimal time of day varies by individual, weather, work, availability of warm water, activities planned after the bath, meals, travel, pūja, visitors and distance from the bathing water.

If the person is healthy and has a long day ahead, Āyurveda advises rising before dawn and bathing immediately to wake up and get started. After bath rituals, the person is clean and ready for the day. Yogis commonly bathe in the river at dawn as it frees them to sit for long mornings of meditation and pūja. Office workers and professionals spending a majority of the day away from home shower early, as they work near strangers and must be clean and smell good. Factory labourers and farmworkers, on the other hand, often need not look clean in the morning, but will want to bathe after a day of dirty work before resting at the day's end. Doctors and cooks should start work with a clean body; they often encounter contamination and shower twice a day—before and after work.

People who work at home have more options. In the winter, many people wait until midday when the air temperature is warmer and more comfortable. In most of the world, where hot water is not readily available, waiting until midday when the sun heats a pail or tank of water is the usual practice. In the West, where hot water is always available, bath time can be any time, and many rituals are made to enjoy the bathtub, including hot tubs, bubble baths, bathhouses, pool parties and romantic dinners in the tub.

While Āyurveda seems unwieldy with many variables determining each instruction, several constants allow universal application of its principles. The consistency of Āyurveda lies in its prescriptions aligning a person with the laws of nature as summarized by the principles of *vāta, pitta, kapha, āma* and *agni.*

Each prescription is designed to alter imbalances by first analysing a patient's nature and then reducing *vāta, pitta* and *kapha* based on the *guna*s of the prescribed substance, activity or medicine.

Part III:
The Bath

~ • 17 • ~

Oil Massage

As tiny tots, my sister and I spent almost every sunny afternoon frolicking naked on the patio. At bath time, one of our elders or designated nanny began by pulling us into the kitchen. Completely unclothing us, she would sit us on the marble floor next to a brass bowl filled with mustard oil and turmeric. The first step to a bath was to get oiled up. This oil would first be massaged onto the top of our heads, then faces, ears, hair, necks and slowly work its way down our limbs, under feet, then the trunks and backs, inspecting each part as it was kneaded. We were then sent out to the high-walled marble verandah to bake in the sun, especially in winter to ward off the phlegmy, mucous-filled ails of the *kapha* winter season.

After our skin was hot, by which time many tiny oily yellow handprints and footprints would coincidentally dot the verandah floor and walls, we would be taken inside. If we itched anywhere, it would be rubbed with a dry herbal powder, usually sharp in odour and made of neem or babul. On Sundays, my aunt would inspect our nails, clipping with tiny surgical scissors.

Finally, our slippery bodies would be carefully transported to the bathroom. Water warmed in the sun in metal pails was used to rinse our little squirming bodies. Green ground *mung* dal paste was applied to remove any excess oil and kneaded into our hair as we tussled with the kneader. Our heads would be rinsed with cool water from another bucket until we were clean, non-gritty and shivering. Finally, a sun-drenched warm towel would come to hug us with a smile.

❧

Oil is widely respected in Āyurveda. Unlike its disastrous reputation in the West for being a killer and contributor to major diseases, oil is much better understood as a vital medicinal agent by Āyurvedists, who treat oils as medicinal substances that must be procured, prepared, stored and used properly.

Known as *sneha*, this Sanskrit term describes the oily, smooth, flowing and heavy properties of oils, fats and ghee, which lend them stability and lubricant properties. Āyurveda describes the importance of different types of oils, upholding sesame oil, ghee, coconut oil and mustard oil as most important. Sesame oil generally calms the dry, rough nature of imbalanced *vāta* and *pitta*. Ghee rebalances all three *dosha*s when used in quantities appropriate to the healthy fire in the body as it can both douse a fire and be digested by it.

Coconut oil is generally cooling and serves as an excellent medium for lowering the inflammatory state of *pitta*. It is commonly used in hot climates, such as in south India. It is applied to oil-rich parts of the body that function optimally at cooler temperatures. Mustard oil, with its sharp and hot nature, rebalances *kapha* and its severe state called *kleda* by cutting through its stagnant, cool and phlegmy nature. Mustard oil is great for kids in the *kapha* stage of life when their baby fat and mucous make them prone to fungal infections.

Modern chemistry recently revealed the dicey nature of overheated oils, in which the long microscopic carbon chains that define fats change from straight chains (cis-fats) into kinked chains (trans-fats). Ancient Indian chemistry classified oils by how long and hard they were cooked. Oils cooked in soft heat for less time were called *mrdu-paka* and could be eaten in small amounts appropriately as food, medicine or *nasya*. Oils not properly cooked, which still contained water or were of a heterogeneous constitution, were called *āma-paka*, because they could produce toxins in the body and were not cooked enough to render them medicinal. Overcooked oil, known as *dgdha-paka*, was indigestible in nature and had no medicinal potency. It was known as *agnimandya*, because it would lower the body's digestive fire and capacity; the excess heating was known to reduce interactive and therapeutic potential. Only the oils cooked for intermediate times or at just the right intensity, *madhya-paka* and *khara-paka*, were used for body massage and certain medicinal applications.

Ancient Āyurveda also prescribed specifically how to handle oils from soil to spoon. It advised which soils and climates produced the best seeds from which oils could be squeezed, and which seasons to grow and pick in. Instructions were given for shelf-life, and how to combine herbs into decoctions before adding to oil, then how to cook the oil and how to know when it had absorbed the correct amount of heat that was needed for the desired application. Because of this, Āyurvedists did not fear oil and its risk for sticking to the body's blood vessels, liver or tissues.

snēhābhyaṅgādyathā-kumbhaścarma-snēhavimardanāt|
bhavatyupāṅgādakṣaśca-dr̥ḍhaḥ-klēśasahō-yathā||85||
tathā-śarīramabhyaṅgāddr̥ḍha-sutvak-ca-jāyatē|
praśāntamārutābādhaṁ-klēśavyāyāmasaṁsaham||86||

Caraka Samhita,
Sūtra-sthāna; chapter 5, slokas 85–86

Just as a pitcher, the dry skin of the body, and an axis of a cart become strong and resistant through the regular application of oil, so by the massage of oil the whole human body becomes strong and the skin smooth. It becomes non-susceptible to diseases of *vāta* and resistant to exhaustion and exertion.

The ancient ritual of starting the bathing process with a coating of oil had three main purposes. Oil penetrates the skin with a coating that pulls out oily dirt, as detergents do. It coats the skin with a smooth, oily shell that counters water—which is drying and sharp—and also fortifies the durable nature of the skin and tissues, which are moist and oily by nature when they are strong and supple. It lowers the dry, rough qualities of excess *vāta* and pacifies the *vāta* that is responsible for pain. It helps hair grow firm and strong in their roots. Oil also speeds up the healing of wounds, burns and rashes on the skin, as it contributes components needed to repair skin tissue.

- Use oil heated at just the right temperature and for the right time to remove oily dirt, counter dryness and fortify the skin and tissues.
- Sesame, the king of oils, is excellent for older people, *vāta* afflictions, and the season of windy cold just before the winter.
- Coconut oil has a cooling effect and lowers *pitta*.
- Mustard oil is sharp and hot in nature and rebalances *kapha*. It is great for kids in the *kapha* stage of life when their baby fat and mucous make them prone to fungal infections.

❧

As the Western, urban and modern lifestyle whirls forward with its productivity, whimsical shopping and easily disconnected relationships (think *vāta*), people notice their hands and legs are dry. They quickly apply hand sanitizer, and when the 62 per cent ethyl alcohol dries, they notice their hands dry again, so they apply a thick lotion. They apply lotion after baths. They apply creams, lotions, gel, foams, ointments and glycerin but are wary to apply pure oil 'because it stains the clothes'.

Lotions trap oil but also trap chemicals in the lotion. Soon, the skin feels drier or develops cracks, redness or rash. The solution is usually a thicker cream or a medicated ointment, which contains prednisones, powerful anti-inflammatory chemicals or antibiotics. The bacteria only penetrated in the first place because there were cracks in the skin from all the drying of the alcohol. The antibiotic cream then kills all the native bacteria that normally live on the skin to prevent worse bacteria from the environment from taking residence. It is a cycle that results in chronic skin irritation or infection. And it is a cycle that is rarely remedied by using medicinal oils.

- Avoid lotions and sanitizers that contain alcohol and trap oil and chemicals in the skin.

Lipid is chemistry lingo for fat. It includes all slippery things in liquid or solid form. Detergents, soaps and cleaners are slippery because of these lipid fats and are used to trap chemicals into balls of fat (like bubbles) and then pull them out of the place where they are hiding, such as the skin, clothes or non-slippery surfaces. They are ideal cleaners. An entire industry of petroleum-based cleaners has emerged from leftover oils that cannot be used in gasoline or petrol. It goes into making plastics, cleansers and some medicines.

Āyurveda prefers to use fats derived from plants and live animals, because it endorses a biological force that processes fats differently when they are in living, organic environments. It prefers plant oils, bone marrow juice and ghee from the milk of animals. Because these fats are synthesized by enzymes in living beings, they are more likely to be metabolized optimally by the human body. Āyurveda tested this logic, experimenting with plant oils in food, medicine and medicinal preparations, keenly observing patients as they applied their theories of *vāta*, *pitta* and *kapha*. Observations were tested and discussed among groups of physicians before they were recorded in textbooks.

For this reason, Āyurvedic physicians trust oils more than synthetic fats and new vegetable oils, such as canola (which is actually rapeseed oil), safflower, mixed vegetable or genetically modified corn oil or peanut oil.

❧ Opt for natural oils pressed from plants rather than those created as byproducts of petrol and gasoline.

At my first Āyurveda class in a yoga studio, the vaidya watched a student lather lotion onto her dry hands during class. He asked humorously, 'Are you going to eat that lotion next?' She quickly frowned and answered, 'Of course not. I would get sick; it is probably poisonous.' To this, the vaidya quickly quipped, 'Then why do you put it on your skin. Doesn't your skin eat?'

This led into an eye-opening discussion on transdermal medicines, such as nitroglycerin patches, nicotine patches, birth control patches and pain medicine patches. We had all heard about the quick delivery of transdermal medicines and how their oil-based formulas allowed chemicals to penetrate through the fat layers of our skin.

In recent years, science has elucidated another pathway into the body apart from blood—the skin. The existence of lymph and nerves was always known and so was the lipid bilayer composing every cell membrane. A network of channels was recently discovered coursing along the highways insulating nerve cells. Information through chemical signals, as well as medicines stored in fat bubbles, is quickly transported through these highways. Experiments have shown that radioactive compounds linked to medicinal drugs cooked into oils that are applied to the skin, especially on the head and back, show up days later inside the deepest fluid pockets of the brain and spinal cord. This generated powerful validation for Āyurvedic oil-based massage therapies and clinical evidence from Āyurvedic *panchakarma* hospitals, where spinal problems and neurological diseases are confidently and competently treated. Lotions and soaps are forbidden there unless they are medicinally prepared. Without the added toxins of the synthetic chemicals, the body gets to business, invoking its healing powers through biologically suitable oil.

❧ Remember, we eat through our skin. If you would not put it in your mouth, do not put it on your skin.

The first time I experienced *abhyanga* in Kerala I wept from the loving kindness of the therapists. *Abhyanga* is an oil massage of the body along Āyurvedic principles. Four women came into my room, gently unclothed me and placed me on a hard neem table, poured hot oil first on my head, then face, neck, back and under my feet. Then, they laid me down on the table face up and each stood in front of one limb. Taking hot oil in unison and in synchronized strokes, they moved from the trunk to the nails in outward strokes, massaging and kneading in sweeps. They moved me to a new position every so often, maintaining their synchronization and their kind but firm touch. For several days in sequence, they worked on me, using slightly different combinations of strokes but each time synchronized and firm to touch certain points.

Gatra mardana, or kneading of the limbs with oil, is an essential step in the bathing process. In addition to helping the oil penetrate the skin, it also presses into the tissues and releases toxins such as lactic acid and trapped old oils and chemicals that may have seeped in. Āyurveda says that a stick dipped into oil and massaged daily will become so supple and strong that it can be bent but not broken. It says that body that is then subject to injury or strenuous work will not be injured, and that the onslaught of aging caused by loss of tone of the skin and muscles will be halted.

Many patients tell me they cannot afford the time or money for massages. Self-massage is also described in Āyurveda as an important art. It keeps the hands strong and makes sure we are familiar with our own bodies. It teaches us how to judge the temperature of hot oil and demands we maintain some vigilance over our body 'as a charioteer has duty towards his chariot.' The three main strokes to learn are *anuloma*, along the lines of the hair, usually outward; *pratiloma*, against the lines of the hair, usually towards the body; and circular, to be done around the elbows, shoulders, knees and heels.

- Massage helps the oil penetrate the skin, presses into the tissues and releases toxins such as lactic acid and trapped old oils and chemicals that may have seeped in.
- Self-massage is just as effective and keeps the hands strong.
- The three main are *anuloma,* along the lines of the hair; *pratiloma*, against the lines of the hair; and circular, to be done around the elbows, shoulders, knees and heels.

Periodically, my aunts would get together for their oil rituals. They would wear sleeveless old nighties and rub each other with mustard or coconut oil. Then, fragrant powder would emerge. It would be placed in a bowl, and my aunts would in turn take each other's arms and rub the powder vigorously along the oiled arm, usually focusing on the flabby pockets that jiggled as they were kneaded. After the heat built up and could no longer be tolerated, they switched to another arm, continuing for several rounds on each person until the oil was gone and the arms and legs were hot. Then they would rise in turn and bathe.

Udvartanam is the use of abrasive powders to remove fat. Due to their dry, rough form and fragrant herbal essential oils, they seep through the base oil applied to the skin to penetrate the *kapha* nature of the fat, breaking it up and slowly removing it over time. There are various subtypes of *udvartanam*, based on ingredients and their effect on *dosha*s. *Utsadana* is a mixture of oil and powder paste that is rubbed on the body to exfoliate and enhance its glow. It is commonly done before weddings or auspicious showy occasions. *Udgharshana* is similar but works through a powder that effectively dries the body to rid it of excess water. It is used more often as a medicine for skin conditions caused by water-retaining irritants and toxins trapped in the skin. Often, skin cloth is also used to enhance action through electrical charges induced by dryness.

There are contraindications to oiling the body. Āyurveda advises that it is dangerous to oil it when the digestive fire, or *agni*, is not balanced. This is because oil clogs the channels for a period of time and will douse fire that is already imbalanced. The *kapha* nature of oil, with its slow, stagnant and cooling tendencies, further lowers the body's fire, making a person lethargic and perhaps destroying their appetite. Exercise is therefore recommended after applying oil, as it opens channels and pores for sweat, centralizes the *agni* and helps pull out toxins, returning the body to its light, energetic, revitalized and optimal state of being.

❧

~ • 18 • ~

Vyayam: Exercise

Babi would emerge from the bathroom in Santoshpur wearing a pair of old navy tennis shorts that could never be worn in public in India. With a smile on his face, and his bare-chested body a shiny yellow-brown, he would begin a strong, brisk walk around the length of the 4000-square-foot flat. After some time, he would stand in one of the bedrooms and begin squatting exercises, bends and warm ups commonly seen on a sports field. Next, he would put a cotton towel around his neck and complete a brisk walk on the wrap-around terrace. Returning, he would check for a mild sweat on his brow and then re-enter the bathroom to take a bath.

My mother's grandfather had a routine *vyayam* as well. He would oil his body at home on Debnathpura Lane in Varanasi. Wearing a dhoti and carrying a cotton towel and fresh dhoti, he would wind through the narrow alleys of the famous ancient city and make his way in the heat to the ghats of the Ganga. There, he would descend the 50–60 stairs and complete his stretches, and then enter the river waters for his daily bath.

While the act of massage helps oils penetrate into the skin and release some of the oil-soluble toxins lying dormant below, the best way to coax toxins out of the layers is to move the body. Exercise creates heat in the body, liquefying oily toxins and drawing them out. It also increases circulation, opening fine capillaries near the surface of the body which carry blood from deep locations up into the skin and out of the body. Exercise also opens the pores and channels through which skin-bound toxins can be released through sweat.

There are three types of exercise: aerobic, those to build resistance and those for flexibility. All three types balance *pitta* and *kapha*. They also rebalance *vāta*, though excess aerobic exercise can aggravate it too. Exercise is known to increase the size of the hippocampus, the brain structure responsible for memory. Psychological tests for memory show significant improvement after exercise, possibly due to increased circulation and oxygen delivery to the brain and possibly due to improved mood. Exercise also improves neuroplasticity, the ability of brain cells to regenerate and alter cell functions in line with the needs of the body.

Aerobic exercise is movement that uses oxygen and lung power. It usually gets the cardiopulmonary system moving and is known to burn calories and fat. Resistance training is exercise that stresses the muscles, forcing work against resistance of weight to build muscle volume and increase strength. Flexibility exercises stretch the muscles, tendons, ligaments and their attachments so that the body has a greater range of motion, is more supple and therefore, is less prone to tears and fractures. All three types of exercise are good for pre-bath *vyayam*.

lāghavaṁ-karmasāmarthyaṁ-diptō-agnirmedasah:-ksaya: |
vibhaktaghanagātratvam-vyāyāmādupajāyatē||

The practice of physical exercise renders the body light and efficient in activities, improves digestive power, decreases obesity, renders finely chiselled contours and consistency in body structure.

Astanga Hrdayam,
Sūtra-sthāna; chapter 2, sloka 11

Exercise is therefore recommended after applying oil, as it opens channels and pores for sweat, centralizes the *agni* and helps pull out toxins, returning the body to its light, energetic, revitalized and optimal state of being.

- Exercise after oiling the body is essential as it opens channels and pores for sweat, centralizes the *agni* and helps get rid of toxins.

❧

~ • 19 • ~

Pranayama: Conscious Breathing

Even as my Babi sits in the house in Princeton, paralysed from his stroke, his lungs are just fine. When he gets frustrated, indeed angry, at the things his body will no longer let him do, his lungs can fuel screams audible to the whole neighbourhood. There is little indication from the volume that his body has been damaged.

Each day as part of his bathing routine, once he has settled into his bathroom, using one arm to undress, he balances himself and slowly sits on a chair in the bathroom. He takes the warmed oil my mother has placed in the same brass bowl he used in Santoshpur and slowly massages it into his left arm, both legs, body and neck, and then calls my mother to massage his back and right arm. My mother watches his slippery body do as much exercise as he can, then his *pranayama*, starting with several rounds of *bhastrika* and *kapalabhati,* and finally a series of *anulom-vilom* as *nadi-sodhana.* If I stand outside the bathroom door, I can often hear him at his breathing exercises, just as I would hear him decades ago in India when I was a curious child watching his every routine. Only when he has completed his exercises will he slowly rise and turn on the water to begin his shower.

With all the effort required just to bathe properly, I wondered for years why he takes the time to do yoga when his body is failing him. He does his *pranayama*, my mother states quietly, because cleaning the lungs is an essential part of bathing the entire body. 'Westerners just sterilize the skin on the outside with soap and water, thinking this makes them clean,' she says. In between, they have chronic odour emanating from their orifices. They do not actually think about cleaning the body through the skin and lungs. They also do not support the skin's need for suppleness and strength by fortifying it. Perhaps that is why they do not make vitamin D as easily any more. And they do not exercise and open the pores before bathing. They do not clean out the lungs or properly scrub the orifices of the body before rinsing everything with water. *Pranayama* is the best way to simultaneously clean out the lungs and send oily toxins out through the open pores as we sweat. Babi breathes before bathing to remind himself of the power of *prana*.

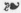

The basic *pranayama* forms can be learnt in a good yoga class. *Bhastrika*, or bellows breath, is a sustained conscious inhale, ending in a hold called the *kumbha*, followed by a conscious sustained exhale ending in *kumbha*. *Bhastrika* maximizes the volume of air held in the lungs and the maximum speed to push it out, exercising the diaphragm and the pleural sac around the lungs.

Kapalabhati literally mean glow (*bhati*) along the forehead (*kapala*), emphasizing the fine beads of sweat that should develop after a round of fast-paced *kapalabhati* breathing. *Nadi-sodhana* means cleaning of the channels and refers to the nasal passages. *Anulom-vilom* describes the flow of air into one nostril and out the opposite one, using the guidance of a finger to block one nostril alternately. *Ujjaya* tightens the vocal cords into a *bandha* or lock, and forces air through, toning the muscles of the larynx. *Sheetali* and *sitkari* are the cooling breaths that draw air flow into the back of the mouth at the palate, just under the pituitary gland. *Bhramhari* is the bumblebee *pranayama* that controls the breath with all the head's orifices blocked except the nostrils, causing an ultrasound effect inside the skull and releasing mucous and phlegm. When practised regularly, *pranayama* improves circulation and stamina.

❧ Before showering or bathing, try doing a round of intense breathing exercises, such as *kapalabhati*. Throw out the inner toxins before cleansing the outer toxins.

❧

~ • 20 • ~

Vegas: The Urges of the Body

Throughout the neighbourhood, we could judge a household's routine just by listening to the body sounds emanating from the house. In my childhood mornings, we would hear the gagging during tongue scraping and gargling in the bathroom with its characteristic echoes, followed by the flow of water. We would hear buckets filling with water before the morning school rush. Occasionally, the sounds of a baby crying, someone with an uncontrolled loud sneeze, spastic belly or large burps after lunch as dishes were gathered would resonate through the air.

These were signals that people were alive and living uninhibited lives. In contrast, life in the land of freedom was more repressed. After we moved to the US, Babi initially changed his routine to fit in with the new culture. My mother would occasionally remind him if he made loud gargling noises, or gagged as he scraped his tongue or belched after a meal. After a couple of years, we moved out of the apartment complex and into a house with a large back yard and plenty of room between houses. Since then, we maintained some distance from the neighbours, in order to preserve our freedom without criticism to 'sing in the shower' and freely release the rest of our body's flows.

❧

Āyurveda describes spontaneous flows through the body that align with subtle impulses in the mind, called urges. Repression of these manifestations of *vāta* leads to imbalances then diseases.

The *saririka* or physical bodily urges, initiated mainly by directed *vāta* flowing out of the body, are called *adharaniya (a* = not; *dharan* = to hold*) vegās*, because they cannot be held back easily. The *manasika*, or psychological urges, are to be self-examined and not expressed, using voluntary control (*dharaniya*) for the sake of spiritual evolution and society's well-being.

Each of the thirteen physical urges is not to be stifled for specific reasons. Called *vegās*, these spontaneously emanate from the body and are part of the body's metabolism and need for waste or *mala*s to be removed from the body. Without these flows, toxins develop.

Urination	Vomiting	Yawning	Tears
Bowel movement	Sneezing	Hunger	Sleep
Sexual release	Belching/Burping	Thirst	Panting
Passing gas			

Caraka Samhita,
Sūtra-sthāna; chapter 7, slokas 3–4

These bodily urges are each associated with nerves and impulses provoked by air, liquid or solid pressing on a canal in the body. For example, when gases from bacteria or chemical reactions in the gut build up, they first distend the gut and then push to escape outward either by moving up or down.

The flows of the body are signals to push things along, mainly the *apana vayu* (downward and outward flow in the body through the pelvis) and *udana vayu* (upward and outward flow from the body through the throat). To resist an urge or create an urge forcefully aggravates *vāta*. Awareness of these urges helps a person avoid the things that will trigger their abnormal expression. In yoga class, we learn how to use our arms and body to recondition the flow of *prana vayu* and *apana vayu* in the correct harmonious directions.

Vegas are controlled by subtle impulses of the mind. These are a collection of signals from all parts of the body that coalesce to alert the unconscious mind that some reflex movement in the body is required. In the nasal cavity, sinuses and throat, when a threshold of chemicals stimulate the receptors, irritation signals accumulate and cause firing together for the contraction of several muscles in the face, depression of the tongue, contraction of the diaphragm and opening of the nostrils to force air through the nose and mouth . . . in what is called a sneeze. This *vegā* is a natural urge created to rid the air passage of that irritant, whether it is pollen, poison or pepper. When people suppress the sneeze, they increase pressure into the closed mouth and nose, and trap those particles back into the passageway. Over time, those particles burrow into the lining of the cavity and create inflammation.

There are three important lasso-type muscles at the bottom of the pelvis, which control the sphincters of excretion. When the lower intestines get filled or the colon begins to rustle, a combination of the gastrocolic reflex, pressure in the rectum, irritation of the nerves and pressure on the sphincters creates the urge to go to the toilet. A similar collection of stimuli create the urge to go empty our urinary bladder.

Āyurveda warned that diseases can transpire if *vegās* are habitually suppressed or forcefully induced over a long period. The diseases may seem to have no direct bearing up on the organ system involved, but these will correspond to where the *vegā* had been aggravated at another time in life.

Many of my patients who had shift work jobs earlier in life were not permitted to go to the toilet when they felt the urge. They held their urges until official breaks were given, in order to prevent interruptions in their work. Years later, many of them complain of incontinence or constipation. They wear adult diapers, are forced to quit their jobs or transfer to less-demanding work schedules. This malfunction of the voluntary muscles to control the bowel or bladder is simply written off as a neurological malfunction 'that just happens' according to modern medicine.

Āyurvedic guidelines suggests optimal times for several *vegās*. These indicate whether we are in optimal flow states. Early morning is the time for the *vegā* to empty our bowels and bladder because toxins and wastes have accumulated overnight. The *kapha* period of 8–9 a.m. is the optimal time for the *vegā* of hunger, and 11.30 a.m.–1.30 p.m. is the optimal time for the *vegā* of midday hunger. If we mindfully allow the body's flows to happen when they happen, healthy bodies will indeed feel urges at these prescribed times of day.

But when our bodies are not in perfect health, our bowels will call to us at different times of day. This should not be ignored, though it may not be convenient for our schedule. As we pay attention to our body and learn its messages through its patterns of flow, we will learn to make the adjustments that will reorient us to the optimal state of health.

The logic of Āyurveda states that flows of the body integrate a number of synchronized muscle and hormonal movements. Conscious suppression of urges over time muddles these automatic orchestrated responses. Āyurveda treats these disorders by simply re-orienting flow, lowering the *vāta* aggravation in that part of the body using herbs, yoga, diet and *vāta*-pacifying substances, and invoking the principle of *vāta* as the theme of proper movement. When the micro-currents of aberrant flow are stilled, like eddies of wind caught in an alley, the flow can be reinitiated slowly and smoothly.

Rishis watched wind flow through the forests, where objects occasionally obstructed its flow. They sat at the river edge and observed water move objects along the main stream and banks and sat at the foothills and watched clouds interact with the mountain tops. This is how they inferred the flow of currents in the universe. Using inference (*anumana* in Sanskrit) and analogy (*upamana* in Sanskrit) to understand flows in nature as similar to flows in the body provided logic and remains among the pillars of evidence-based medicine in Āyurveda. As in the macrocosm, so in the microcosm.

Do not ignore or suppress these urges:

- Urination, bowel movements, sexual release, passing gas, vomiting, sneezing, belching/burping, yawning, hunger, thirst, tears, sleep and panting.

~ • 21 • ~

Skin and Nails

Every Sunday, my Babi would call me to him, somewhere between my mother's rituals with me and my sisters. He would hand me a large nail clipper and ask me to cut and file his toenails. He liked the way I observed the nail bed and inspected each nail in its home before I cut and shaped it so that it would not damage his socks. I would then oil Babi's nails and toes, massaging each one to improve circulation. Then I would move up to his hands, doing the same with care and a sense privilege for getting to sit so close and spend time with him. Once I had asked why Sunday morning was the appointed time for such a task: I had seen my teacher clipping her nails regularly during our study period as she sat at her desk. My mother told me that Sunday mornings were the day of the sun and a day of calm and self-care.

Now, Babi is older but his nails are not frail. On Sundays, he still looks at me, but now sheepishly. I take the same hand that could lift me with one sweep and place me on top of his shoulder, and look at his strong, hard nails; strong and hard like his determination. I meander through tear-filled memories and compassion for this genius of a man who is trapped in his beautiful strong body, and push aside tear-jolting anger at the self-neglect that ambition creates, often landing people in conditions such as paralysis. In between, my hands automatically take the same large nail clipper that was gifted to him in Cambridge and begin with his toes, observing, inspecting, cutting and shaping, oiling and massaging before moving up to his hands. After I finish, he rises slowly and heads toward the bathroom for his shower.

❧

The *dhatu*s of Āyurveda describe physiology and the formation of tissues of the body. Just as modern science saw embryos develop, so did the ancient *rishi*s, but they interpreted the same data differently due to a different world view. This is the root of the difference between modern medicine and Āyurveda. In the Āyurvedic world view, energies that become heavy precipitate from fast-flowing energy into particles or substances, and become matter. The physical expression of the energy being is the body. If the energy being is a constellation of *dosha*s, the physical expression of that constellation is the precipitate of *dhatu*s, the tissues of the body.

According to *dhatu* theory, the body is composed of seven tissue types, all interconnected and all interdependent. When one tissue is not formed properly, the subsequent tissues lose their strength. The *mamsa dhatu*, approximate to muscle tissue, is thought to arise from *rakta dhatu*, the nourishing fluid energy circulating in blood. As the muscle tissue develops, the leftover building blocks are used to make the coatings over the muscles, known as skin. Watch a growing baby bird. Only after its muscles are fully developed will a translucent sheen slowly solidify into its skin.

Āyurveda proposes that since the skin is an outgrowth (*upadhatu)* of muscle tissue, all diseases of the skin are rooted in that which makes *mamsa dhatu*. Simply put, Āyurveda connects all outer skin diseases to the blood and muscle that feed it from the gut.

In modern anatomy too, the root (*mula*) of skin is the embryonic mesoderm, a middle layer of tissue in the body that develops into the gut. Āyurveda substantiates its theory with patients in whom the skin healed after the gut healed. When the gut is unhealthy, symptoms appear on the skin. Over time, chronic skin problems, such as psoriasis, vitiligo, rosacea and eczema, are healed by altering the gut's flow and function, emphasizing medicines by mouth over topical treatments. Based on this, Āyurveda concluded that the skin on the outside is connected to the skin on the inside. Visit any good Āyurvedic physician today with a skin problem, and she/he will ask you about your diet, your bowel movements and your appetite.

In contrast, *dhatu* theory considers nails as outgrowths of *asthi-dhatu*, approximate to bone tissue, whose leftover unusable building blocks called *mala*s form hard shells. According to Āyurveda, when the *asthi-dhatu* is not healthy, it shows up as problems and weakness in hair and nails.

This was a strong influence in my relationship to nail polish. As a child, my mother would apply nail polish for us only once a month or on special occasions, using one light coat and not permitting any sealants or fixants. She did not allow us to cut our cuticles, insisting that nail polish should not harm the inner body. In a week, with the wear and tear of young girls' lives, the nail polish would chip off. We would have to wait for the next coating. In the meantime, she would encourage us to apply oil and ghee to the nails. From college, I worked in a laboratory where university regulations did not permit the use of nail polish on the fingers for lab workers. This continued during medical school, where we scrubbed into surgeries; nail polish was forbidden.

Seeking cosmetic solace after I became a full-fledged physician, I began to paint my toenails one summer. Soon thereafter, I noticed that my hair began to fall out and my nails became weak. I attributed it to stress and ignored the whispered echoes from childhood. Finally, I discontinued using nail polish, noticing that the nails looked dull in the few moments between cleaning off an old coat of polish and applying a new one. I allowed the nail to stay without polish for a few days and applied ghee to my toes and fingernails, massaging it into the nailbeds. Within a week, I noticed small new hairs growing at the scalp. Perhaps a coincidence, the scientist in me might say. But over months, I noticed the natural sheen return to my nails and the parting on my scalp become narrower.

One day, a successful self-made colleague announced that she was becoming an entrepreneur and starting her own natural cosmetics line. From her background, I knew she could be successful, as she had worked for personal products lines and knew how to market many self-care products. She confided her biggest challenge: all the available data showed there was no non-toxic nail polish. For months, she searched for ingredients that would stick to the nails permanently, but could be removed. She called me one day and announced she would no longer be wearing nail polish. She found data that showed correlation with hair breakage, as well as teratogenicity, the ability to harm an unborn child. Toluene, methacrylates and phthalates were at the top of the list as known teratogens, mostly through inhalation and small vapourized particles that landed on the body or touched the nailbed skin chronically, but the implications of the data were that harm was possible.

Āyurveda predicts weakened bones and hair when nail polish is usually regularly. Nail polish—which contains chemical synthetic ingredients to harden it, maintain colour and provide flexibility and shine—is known to be toxic when inhaled or absorbed through the skin. If nails can absorb oil, they can absorb chemicals over time.

- ❧ Oil and massage nails to make them stronger.
- ❧ Avoid nail polish, because if nails can absorb oil, they can absorb chemicals too.

☙

Mudras are hand postures with coded meaning. Like sign language, mudras developed to accompany dance, meditation, yoga and *japa*, the repeated evocation of mantras. There are twenty-eight main mudras used in dance, as outlined in the *Hasta-bina-ya*, or hand gestures, of the Natya Shastra, an authoritative dance text believed to written circa 800 CE. In total, there are twenty-four *asaṁyuta* (separated, that is, one-handed gestures) and thirteen *saṁyuta* (joined, that is, two-handed gestures) mudras. The Abhinaya Darpana, by the sage Nandikesvara, written circa 5th century CE, studies a multitude of aspects of theatre and dance, including facial movements and hand gestures, and outlines twenty-eight root mudras.

When done properly, it is believed that hand gestures code meaning in the brain and aid meditation. For example, the *gyana mudra*, which aids in the psychic connection to knowledge, is made by joining the edge of the pointer finger to the edge of the thumb to make a circle, and extending the remaining three fingers outward, keeping a flat palm. It is thought to increase clear *vayu* or air quality around the person's mind, allowing it to relax and thus focus on meditation.

Many mudras accompany yoga poses just before meditation, such as the *vaayu mudra*, the chin mudra, the *prana mudra* and the *surya mudra*. They have specific indications and effects that were confirmed by thousands of people such that they remained in classic texts as current, relevant information for health and well-being.

☙

~ • 22 • ~

Hair

My father has a ponytail. His head is full of hair and only about half of it has turned grey, even though he is seventy-five. His bones and nails are strong. One of his favourite things, which I admit I sometimes do just to pacify him when he is upset about one of my many rebellious acts, is to run my fingers through his hair as he sits trapped in his chair. I massage his scalp and tug handfuls of his long locks strongly for a few seconds. It may seem unusually intimate at this age, but we are Bengali and Indian, and we do not fear loving our elders tenderly. Babi has also always been a glutton for head massages.

Hair tugging is a long tradition in my family. My baby sister used to climb up to me when she was two and give me head massages and gentle hair tugs to help me wake up. I would do the same to her to help her fall asleep. My mother would tug my hair in sections each night as I sat on the floor between her knees before she oiled and braided my hair for sleep each night. My mother would then call me to tug her hair and massage her neck when she was tired or worried, or wanted to connect with me. My memories of our family centre around watching her comb and braid each of our heads before bed, before school and on school picture day. Grooming and hair care was a family affair between aunts, cousins and sisters, and I wonder if we are the only clan in the world that has such an intimate relationship with hair.

❧

Because hair is related to the health of the *asthi-dhatu*, hair is oiled and nourished to keep the bones healthy. It is not treated as waste or an outgrowth, like a hangnail or mucous secretion. Hair provides protection from the sun, warmth to the body, protection from flying particles and mild cushioning from anything that might come near the head.

Āyurveda mentions a few conditions in which oiling of the head is not recommended. It should be avoided when someone is suffering from severe imbalances in *kapha*, in which mucous and the qualities of oil are disturbed in the body. This includes severe and phlegmy head colds, infections, sinusitis and inflammatory problems in the head and neck, severe lung problems, extremely oily skin, lipid disorders, obesity, initial stages of fever and indigestion. People just completing *panchakarma* purifications and purges also should not oil the head. The logic behind these prohibitions is that oil, which is *kapha* in nature, is converted to unhealthy *kapha* and adds to that already present in the body, furthering the condition.

❧ Do not oil your head if you have a severe or phlegmy head cold, infection in the head and neck, sinusitis or severe lung problems, extremely oily skin, lipid disorders, obesity, initial stages of fever or indigestion, as it may further the condition.

❧

In one of her lighter speeches in the 1990s as First Lady, Hillary Clinton, not yet a Senator or Secretary of State, gave a speech about the all-important topic of hair. She began with tales of her experiments with hairstyle choices day to day, just as people change their outfits and shoes. She revealed the uneasiness of people around her as she varied her hairstyles. Her appearance changed significantly with different cuts, despite the same blonde colour due to the drastic altered reflections of mood, gravity and poise.

She discussed consistency. When we change our style frequently, people cannot decide who we are, and it makes them uncomfortable. She emphasized the importance of hair in framing the face, in presenting oneself culturally, sexually and politically, and in choosing how we want to be seen.

- Keep hair healthy and clean. It will reflect your inner strength, no matter how you choose to style it.
- Consider the importance of consistency in your life and what your hairstyle reflects about you in your work and cultural environment.

The concept of shampoo derives from the Sanskrit root *capayati,* which means to press and knead with the intention of soothing. A similar word *chāmpo* in Hindi is the imperative of *chāmpnā*, to smear, knead the muscles of the body and oil massage the head and hair. Europeans who travelled as traders to India partook in the rituals of the bath, getting their hair oiled and cleansed with herbal mixtures, rather than perfuming their heads and covering them with wigs.

Cleansing of the hair became a new craze when the practice was introduced to Europe by Bengali barber–surgeon Din Muhammad and his Irish wife Jane Daly, who opened a bathhouse in the 1700s in Brighton, England. Adapting the necessary components, they created shampoo, which is basically a soapy, slippery fat combined with another fat to make a viscous liquid that can be moved around the scalp unlike a bar of soap. Salt is often added to thicken the slippery nature. Fragrance, colour and preservatives are added to modern versions of shampoo.

Herbs commonly used to rinse out oil were green gram powder, powder of the *amalaki* fruit (*Emblica officinalis*), *shikakai* (*Acacia concinna*) or hibiscus flowers. These leave hair soft, shiny and manageable. To spread the powder into thick hair, the fruit pulp of plants containing saponins, natural surfactants, were added. Soapberries, soap nuts that created lather called *phenaka* or extract of boiled sapindus—a tropical pan-Indian tree also called *ksuna*—was added to herbal cleansing powders and applied to the oily head. The ancients also added a plethora of herbs in combinations specifically to either lower unharmonious *vāta*, raise *agni*, improve the quality of digestive fire, transform *pitta* or lower sticky *kapha*, utilizing access to a rich blood supply through the scalp.

~ • 23 • ~

Shaving and Haircut

When we were very little and lived in a joint family with my mother's siblings and my father's nephews, my parents gathered all the kids and men once a month and stood everyone in a line. As they sipped tea and waited their turn, my mother would snip and my father would take an electric razor and trim the napes of each person's neck. Once in a blue moon, someone would have their head shaved. My parents were confident with pageboy cuts, bangs and trims. After each person's cut, they would be rushed off to the bathroom for oiling and a bath.

At the age of twelve, my sister notified me that since we lived in America, we were expected to shave regularly, even as women. She brought me a pink razor and instructed me to run it along my legs and under my arms, just before showering. I was terrified, as I had witnessed blood when men shaved their beards, and my legs and underarms were much softer and much less hairy than their faces. I cried desperately as she forced the razor down my leg, capturing a few wisps. When I told my mother, she told me to apply mustard oil to my legs instead. The heat inherent to mustard oil destroys the hair follicles and makes them less hairy. Religiously, I began to use mustard oil on my legs for several months. To this day, I do not really know if it worked, but I know that very little hair lives there.

Men who shaved in the 1960s know the difference between shaving powder, foam, gel and cream due to the advent of television and all the products that suddenly arose. They also know what a shaving brush is. With the advent of electric razors, safety razors and huge marketing for self-care shaving products, many younger men do not know the multitude of options available decades earlier because their choices are limited to foam and razor.

Copper razors date back to 3000 BCE, and a variety of sharp tools, scissors and trimmers have evolved to meet the religious, cultural and military needs of those who shave. Natural products were gathered to assist in the process of getting the skin and hair ready for the blade and were the norm until forty years ago. Warm water was used to soften the skin around the follicles and the hair for several minutes, and often a soapy or lubricating agent was applied. After the shave, alum, a crystal of potassium, aluminum and sulfate could be applied to stop any bleeding or irritation. An astringent such as aloe would soothe the skin and stop cuts or bleeding. Moisturizing oil or fat would be applied to smooth any irritated skin.

Called *kshaur-karma*, the cutting of hair, shaving and clipping of nails was recommended to be done weekly to increase purity and lessen the effects of age. Shaving was considered part of the cleansing routine and a beautification exercise, but also deeply connected with the mind and soul. Suśruta—the father of ancient surgery, embryology and one of the ancient articulate wise men—who wrote about the structure and function of the human body as its physiology in Varanasi around 1000 BCE, advised that shaving daily alleviates the evil tendencies of the mind, reduces tension and heaviness, and induces a cheerful disposition. He espoused that beard shaving daily energized a man. If a beard was maintained, it required shaping and trimming. Even at that time, it was advised that brushes and razors for cutting hair and nails be kept clean and not shared. Visiting cosmetic shops was not advised, as it increased the chance of impurity in public spaces.

❧

~ • 24 • ~

Cleaning the Feet and Perineum

Each time Babi would return from a long journey, it was my job to sit at his feet and gently take off his wing-tipped shoes and socks, clean his feet, and then later clean and polish his shoes and bring them for inspection. Depending on how tired he was, I would either use a cloth to wipe his feet and inspect his toes and heels, so he could go bathe immediately, or I would ask him whether he wanted the full cleaning. On his nod, I would happily bring a wide basin with warm water, gently roll up his trouser cuffs and soak his feet in the water. Using a brush, a loofah, his nail file and some oil, I would first brush his heels, scrub gently until his soles were smooth and then work on his toes.

His feet were always hard, reflecting his barefoot years as an orphan living on the streets of Calcutta in the 1930s, where he had survived the famines and watched the death of several siblings. My father's feet had walked miles from there to the Sealdah railway station to a train that took him to his destiny. It was an honour to sit at his feet. I would scrub and soothe, gently pad his wet, clean feet and place them on a dry soft towel. Then I would use warm mustard oil and massage his toes, his instep, his soles and his ever-hard heels. During this time, he would talk with the adults around him, telling tales of his latest travels, listen to the things that required his attention on his return or the misadventures of his children and relatives. Occasionally, he would pull back his feet from some sensation or my carelessness. He was rarely ticklish, and I was too timid to test his limits. When the oil had soaked in, he would gesture to me, withdraw his feet and rise to move towards his awaiting oil bowl and bath.

mēdhyaṁ pavitram-āyuṣ-yama-lakṣmī-kali-nāśanam|
pādayōrmalamārgāṇāṁ-śaucādhānamabhīkṣṇaśaḥ||

Āyurveda advises that we frequently clean the feet and excretory orifices with water and earth-made natural substances. Cleaning these lower surfaces of our body promotes intelligence, brings about purity and longevity, and a greater awareness of cleanliness. It eliminates inauspiciousness and the bad effect of Kali.

Caraka Samhita,
Sūtra-sthāna; chapter 5, sloka 98

Both literally and figuratively, our feet are our tangible connection with the planet. When we walk with our feet, or rest them on the ground, we are connected to the subtle energy fields in the earth. While they are minuscule and hardly noticeable, they are indeed present and detectable by seismometers and other subtle magnetometers. To keep this connection as acute and sensitive as possible, the feet should be clean and able to sense pressure, temperature and heat.

Busy people often neglect their heels and insteps. Cracks on the heels signify deep inner *pitta–vāta* imbalance and dryness, usually an indication that the mind is moving too fast and creating some level of chaos in the body. It also implies that the digestive fire is not of optimal transformative quality, and the gut function or mind is out of balance. The solution is to institute *vāta*-pacifying measures into the diet, the lifestyle and the attitude by spending time in meditation, resolving conflicts and changing one's outlook so that calm and peace pervade one's being. This is easier said than done for many, but Āyurveda advises that heel cracks indicate a need for inner harmony.

The instep is a sign of the resilience and flexibility of the body and mind. As we endure difficulties in life and become curmudgeonly, we may find that our instep becomes flatter. Interestingly, though modern medicine provides no definitive cure for flat feet, or plantar fasciitis, Āyurveda recommends a six-week twice-daily course of yoga poses that resurrects the flexibility and strength of the instep. Among them is *utkatasana*, a thirty-second pose standing on the balls of the feet, gradually lowering the body while keeping the heels suspended. Over several days, one can watch the feet become stronger. Patients suffering previously with plantar fasciitis have proven the power of this benign, non-surgical intervention.

- Keep your feet clean and soften the hard outer skin through oiling, paying special attention to the heel and instep.
- *Utkatasana* helps reverse the effects of flat-footedness. To practice, stand on the balls of the feet for 30 seconds, gradually lowering the body while keeping the heels suspended.

As a child, all our letters would begin with *srī-charaneshyu*, translated as the English salutation 'Dear', but literally meaning, 'Respected sir whose feet I touch and remember here . . .' There are many reasons we touch the feet of elders in India, but despite all the variations in different corners and cultures of India, all signify respect and the offering of *pranam*.

Pranam is a complicated concept to explain to a person not familiar with dharma. It conveys respect for the elderly, the wise and those who are admired. Another philosophical version states that by touching feet and then the self, we convey that the lowest part of another person remains higher than our selves. Others say that when we touch the feet of an elder, some of their energy is transferred to our hands, which we then transfer to ourselves. In turn, when the same elders touch the head of a person in blessing, energy is exchanged between them, giving the blessed person mental strength, motivation and vigour.

There are many ways of touching the feet. For some, the student draws close to the teacher and touches the teacher's right foot with the right hand, then the left foot with the left hand. For others, a person touches the shins not the feet to avoid the shoes but touch the person. In other cultures, the right hand is always used, keeping the left hand touching the right forearm as a proxy of using both hands. After contacting the feet, the hands then touch one's forehead and heart, or only the heart, signifying the connection between the person who was touched and the mind of the person offering *pranam*.

Sometimes, instead of touching feet, we give *Brahmānjali*—the offering of divine potential—by putting hollowed hands together and looking at the other person, signifying hands performing virtues reflecting a person's character. It is said that greetings should never be done with one hand only, as the *anjali* is a sign of humility and devotion.

For many, the first people we *pranam* each day are our parents, a reminder that we can never repay the debt we owe them.

❧

Sitting in the Harvard Club, I reflexively remove my sandals and wrap my legs under my hips as I sit on a mahogany chair with encrusted logo in the grand hall. Hurriedly, a gentleman with white gloves comes over to remind me of the rules to leave shoes on and never ever put feet on the furniture. It is one of those moments when two cultures collide in my head, as I politely smile and lower my clean feet into my dirty sandals, while he perceives dirty feet re-entering the solace of proper shoes on his clean floor. Feet and shoes are something we cannot try to convince cultures about.

It is always difficult when I initially return from India, where I reflexively remove my shoes when entering the room, home or office of any respected person. In the US, I am requested to not remove my shoes. 'What a nuisance to see dirty shoes outside the door, where we are welcoming people into our home,' they say, or 'We don't want your smelly socks tracking through our clean carpet.' I quietly put my shoes on, complying with transferring the streets of the US onto their floors.

Āyurveda has a different view. After spending all day walking on the feet, often in sandals or barefoot, they need to be cleaned of dust, grime and sweat. If dust builds up on the feet, they can slowly crack the outer layers and promote cracks and fissures, faster than the exfoliation that regularly repairs the underside of the feet.

As a matter of routine and ritual, Āyurveda advises we wash our feet in the morning after rising, before going to the altar for morning prayer, at the time of bath, before sitting for each meal, at sunset prayer and before bed. In addition, feet should be washed before and after sexual intercourse, entering temples and attending auspicious ceremonies. In traditional Indian settings, most occasions obviously require bare feet and maintenance of clean floors where people sit, such as altar rooms, temples, beds and dining halls. But in the West, people do not usually remove their shoes, so washing the feet becomes a nuisance.

- Wash your feet in the morning after rising, before morning prayers, while bathing, before sitting for each meal, at sunset prayer, before bed, before and after sexual intercourse, entering temples and attending auspicious ceremonies.

My grandmother and her mother-in-law before her, and hers before her, performed an intimate ritual each morning. My mother was notified that this was to be passed down in our lineage through the ages and maintained. At the beginning of the day, before ingesting food, a wife would place a cup formed from her palm and fingers filled with water before her husband's great toe of his right foot. Usually, he would wash his feet first as a sign of respect to her. He would then dip his toe gently into the water. She would then put this hand gently to her lips and drink the water, wiping the residual water in the hand over the back crown of her head, just as holy water is taken.

In the family, this was considered one of the holiest symbols of devotion. If he did not walk cleanly in life and his foot pointed into filth, it would then poison his wife, and the mother of his children would die. If he was not gentle when dipping, it would hurt her, and her broken or neglected heart would not nourish him. As the decades have passed, my mother reminds her four girls of traditions as the debate on marriage as an institution continues.

❧

During the fall semester when I am teaching, a frenetic pace pervades the classroom, keeping people's feet off the ground. Students have just too much going on: appointments, commitments and deadlines. For many years, I resigned it to the nature of academia, but it seemed true in every profession and could be observed even in schoolchildren.

Āyurveda correlated activity with meteorology and the seasons: as the hot weather cools in the weather, *vāta* begins to aggravate. Winds form as a result of movements of hot air rising as cool air descends, while the sun shifts and the plants dwindle in making foliage. The cold, dry and windy weather is matched with a group of fast-moving, fast-talking, doing-too-much, dry-skinned over-achievers.

Vāta pacification is the cure for the monkey mind racing frantically, creating anxiety and mania, and promoting insomnia and nightmares. Regular practices to slow the mind are recommended. For first-timers desperate for help, meditation and yoga are usually not useful. People who practise daily and continue developing tools through the autumn months have excellent grounding and awesome stamina. Shifting from yoga to grounding, slow asanas that are less acrobatic calms unwieldy *vāta*. Quietude is essential. Switching to *vāta*-pacifying food means less cold, dry, light and rough food—less sandwiches, dry fruits, cold coffee and more soups, warm salads, vegetable medleys, rice dishes and warm spices in chai.

Āyurveda suggests warm sesame oil. Lotion is not a substitute, because the skin can drink oil, but lotion has many artificial components that cannot be absorbed by the body. Just before bed, rub warm sesame oil vigorously under the feet, then on top of the feet, behind the ears and at the fontanelle spot on top of the head. Allow the oil to soak in, making note of the time it takes. Very dry bodies with high *vāta* imbalance will soak in the sesame oil within 5 minutes. Less *vāta* imbalanced people will take longer.

You can put a pair of old cotton socks on the feet so that they do not stain your bedsheets or carpet. In the morning, monitor how you feel. Many people report sounder sleep, less nighttime waking, diminished nightmares and a fresher morning. Āyurveda predicts that as *vāta* is pacified, all the functions of the body begin to return to the optimal level.

In winter,

- Switch to slow, grounding asanas and meditation to pacify the mind.
- Eat less cold, dry, light and rough food—such as sandwiches, dry fruits, cold coffee, soups, warm salads, vegetable medleys, rice dishes and warm spices in chai.
- Rub sesame oil under the feet, then on top of the feet, behind the ears and at the fontanelle spot on top of the head. Allow the oil to soak in, making note of the time it takes.

The perineum is that all-important area at the bottom of the pelvis where three muscles hold in the gut and keep everything from falling out. Āyurveda strongly suggests that we use water daily to clean this area, no matter what we have done during the day after excretions. Just before entering the bath, Āyurveda advises we wash our feet, squat down and clean our excretory areas with water and throw that water out, then proceed to a clean water bath.

~ • 25 • ~

Bathing

Hobbling out from his room, Babi is smiling. His pepper-grey hair is wet, and his beard is spreading water along the collar of his shirt. I move closer, to adjust his sweater and close his cuffs and belt properly. I need to feel needed. My father is stubbornly independent, just as he is aware of his increasing frailty and dependence on others to complete his grooming. Until all the steps of his routine are complete, he cannot move to the outer rooms, where unexpected visitors may arrive. He moves with his cane past the full-length mirror and inspects his work. He asks for an adjustment of his socks and then descends the stairs, one by one, satisfied that he has prepared himself to accept another day.

❧

pavitram-vrashyamayushyam-shramaswedamalapaham |
sharira-balasandhanam-snanamojaskaram-param ||

The body is purified by bathing. Bathing enhances libido, and is life-giving. It eliminates fatigue, sweat and dirt. It augments the liveliness and force of the body, giving strength and is one of the best ways to enhance *ojas*.

Caraka Samhita,
Sūtra-sthāna; chapter 5, sloka 94

Medicinally, water on the body, especially if it is cool or cold, closes the pores and capillaries in the skin, thus shifting the blood flow away from the periphery of the body and back to the larger arteries. The trunk, known as the *kostha* or central zone, becomes warmer, and the central heater of the body around the gut focuses the energy toward the digestive system—making the person hungrier. This is why bathing is encouraged before eating a meal—food will digest better when the blood is circulating near the gut.

However, one should not just blindly accept this postulate. Āyurveda encourages us to use *pratyaksha*, or personal experience and observation to validate its advice. Experiment on your own body. On two different days, take a bath at the same time of day. On day one, eat before your bath; on day two, eat after your bath. Decide for yourself how your gut feels and whether your hunger is different.

❧ On one day, eat before bathing. On the second day, eat after bathing. Observe which one you prefer, whether you feel any difference in terms of hunger and digestion.

After several plagues during the Middle Ages of Europe wiped out nearly half of the population between 1100 CE and 1400 CE, people became afraid of water, fearing its nature. Europeans had virtually stopped bathing. Men came hunting for the mythical India, as they had heard of secret potions, healing spices and the philosopher's stone from the Greek book *Indika* on Indian medicines, documented by Ctesias around 400 BCE. Only myths remained in Europe of Indian people who bathed with oil, used healing hospitals and maintained universities—which contained knowledge of healing panaceas—later destroyed by Islamic and Christian conquests.

But even with their arrival in India after their Renaissance, explorers could not absorb the richness of Āyurveda and just took bits of hygiene and comforts back to Europe. They witnessed people bathing in the water and tried it themselves, but could not imagine the waters of Europe allowing the same protection. When they returned to Europe, they did not replicate the ritual of oiling, perhaps because it stained the clothes. They absorbed the idea of immersing themselves in water by inventing large tubs that could hold water and a person. First made of wood, then later of porcelain and shaped oblong, the bathing tub became a phenomenon, symbolizing beauty and sensuality.

The nature of water is dry and sharp. It slowly pulls natural oils from our skin, which is naturally unctuous in its healthy state. That is why Āyurveda advises us to oil our bodies before rinsing with water. Cold air further dries the skin by closing skin pores that slowly secrete oils. Clean oil penetrates through outer skin to remove to bring oily dirt to the surface using light exercise that induces sweat. Then the water can remove dirt and grime.

bhishagyo-bhishaktara-apah |

Water is the best among all medicines.

The Bath: Practical

A traditional bath does not begin with water; it ends with it. The cleaning of the body requires the excess and imbalanced *dosha*s to be coalesced to the outer skin, where soap, detergent, oil or ash can pull it out of the body and away. To do this, a bath begins with an oil massage, a herbal powder rub if needed, exercise to open the pores and increase circulation, *pranayama* to get the breathing and circulation flowing, movement of bodily urges, trimming of hair and nails and cleaning of the feet and excretory surfaces of the body.

Then the rinsing of the body with water can begin. Cold or cool water is best, especially above the collar bones, as the head and neck are filled with fat-drenched structures that will deform in heat. Never ever should very hot water be used for daily showers. When the body is rinsed, a dry clean cotton towel should be used to pat, not harshly wipe, the skin, hair and body, working from the top of the head down the body. After the body is clean, a new day begins.

❧

Part IV: Activities of the Day: Yoga Off the Mat

As the sun rises early in the morning, my mother is on her yoga mat in the grand window room, having pushed aside boxes yawning open in *savasana*. She is committed to her yoga now more than ever because it has cured her arthritis and she no longer creaks with the stairs as she descends them. Babi and I admire her devotion as we sit in the adjacent room, sipping tea.

As I push myself towards the yoga mat, remembering Babi's dedication to teaching me complicated asanas as a young child, the reality strikes that he may never sit again in those postures after this stroke. My waistline signals a secret disease of inertia, resisting exercise and harbouring unprocessed emotions and stress.

After my mother finishes with a loud series of oms, she comes to join us, preparing a glass of hot water boiled with fresh ginger and black pepper. I try to coax her into inspiring me to also sit on the yoga mat because there is a part of me that really does want the exercise. She reminds me that yoga is not only on the mat. 'True yoga is off the mat,' she says. 'It is living life with the mind yoked to the body. Yoga on the mat is just practice yoga. Yoga off the mat is how you live your life.'

❧

Part IV:
Activities of the Day: Yoga Off the Mat

~ • 26 • ~

Sadvritta and Dharma

On the detailed census form that has arrived, my disabled father must complete several demographic questions and return it to the government. For the question on religion, he mumbles, 'They cannot ask that question in a secular society. Tell them *sanatana dharma* and mark the Other box!'

I ponder before filling in the bubble on the form, knowing he is avoiding the word Hindu, not because he does not like Hindus, but because he does not like the way Westerners describe it as a pagan religion worshipping elephants and monkeys.

Sanatana dharma is the world view of eternalism, which aligns a person's life values to the timeless principles of nature. It is the original name of what is now popularly called Hinduism. It explores the principles and science of the forces of nature, which in modern society are called the physical sciences and natural sciences, such as geology, physics, astronomy, chemistry, meteorology, metallurgy and biology. *Sanatana dharma* sees nature and its laws as the backbone of honesty. Truth is the way the clouds, mountains, trees and animals behave. This philosophy was adapted to the human mind, which becomes convoluted and muddy from the ego.

The idea of what is true and right is explored in Western philosophy as epistemology and ontology. Epistemology is the study of the nature and scope of knowledge, known as *veda* in Sanskrit. Ontology is the study of the nature of reality and of being, known as dharma, asking the heavy questions, 'What is real?' and 'What is the meaning of being?'

The term *sanatana dharma* and the idea that the mind could know what is right and real was first mentioned and explained in depth in the Rig Veda, the first of the four classics of Vedic literature, one of the oldest texts created by humankind to understand the world and itself, circa 10,000 BCE. *Sanatana* refers to the eternal and the idea of knowing that which has neither beginning nor end, nor limits and boundaries.

It was the working way of truth and cosmic order with a code of ethics so obvious that it was neither named nor identified by its users until invaders from central Asia described it as the way of life for those living east of the Indus River, or the h-Indus. The term Hinduism began to pervade the literature west of Asia and was even used by the submissive brown gentlemen of the 1700s. Even today, those educated in Western schools call themselves Hindus. In the quest for India's freedom, after suffering enough of Persian and European invaders, a revivalism movement began in order to avoid having to use the term Hindu because of its non-native, Persian origin.

Āyurveda follows the philosophy of *sanatana dharma*, with a medical world view that the body will decay faster when not aligned with truth because it is misaligned from nature. Nature will realign or else destroy all that is not in harmony with it in order to main overall balance.

My mother interprets this when I ask her how to know what is right. 'If I find a pen on the ground, should I pick it up? It does not belong to me, yet to whom does it belong when someone has lost it?' My mother's discernment on conscience is impeccable. She answers simply, as decades of reading the Bhagavad Gita daily and translating Tagore's poems have guided her.

She says that as you see the pen, whatever thought spontaneously manifests in your mind is the correct way. If you have spent time cleaning your mind daily, with meditation and yoga, you will be aligned. If your aligned mind tells you to take the pen, then you should follow that path of karma and choose it as your right way, accepting the consequences of what will happen and not happen due to your picking up the pen and claiming new ownership. It, with all its karmas, will enter your life.

If, however, on seeing the pen, your mind spontaneously tells you that the pen is not yours and that someone dropped it and may come back looking for it, as improbable as it may be, it is your duty to follow your mind's original decree. Live life this way, and you will have no regrets, accept all punishments and enjoy all the bounty that comes to you without guilt that perhaps you did not deserve it.

satyam-vada priyam-vada ma-vada-satyam-apriyam |
priyamapi-na-anritam-vada esha-dharma-sanatana ||

Speak truth, speak it pleasantly, do not speak truth in an unpleasant or unloving manner; even if it is pleasant never speak untruth, this is the *sanatana dharma.*

~Taittiriya Upanishad; petal 5, section 11;
adapted by Manu Smriti (4.138), circa 1250 BCE

❧ In cases of confusion, follow your inner heart's first instinct.

❧

While India has become modern, it is currently engaged in a deep battle, not in the physical world but in the mental plane. The latest challenge and invasion of the subcontinent that suppresses Āyurveda is oppression by Western thought, brought not by men and guns but by advertising, education and philosophy that denies *sanatana dharma*.

Satyameva jayate, now a common slogan in modern India, comes from the ancient proverb, *truth alone prevails*. It is a well-known mantra from the ancient Indian scripture Mundaka Upanishad, 3.1.6. Adopted as the national motto of India at independence, it is inscribed in the Devanagari script at the base of the national emblem, and on the left-hand bottom corner of all Indian currency notes. The emblem is an adaptation of the lion symbol of Ashoka, erected around 250 BCE in Sarnath, just north of Kashi. It was brought into the national lexicon by Pandit Madan Mohan Malaviya in 1918. While serving his second of four terms as President of the Indian National Congress, he also founded Banaras Hindu University to nurture a new generation of scholars devoted to truth.

Principles of self-control and correct action aligned with conscience are known in Āyurveda as *sadvrtta*. The Sanskrit term *sad* or *sat* means truthful, pure or good, depending on context. The Sanskrit term *vrtta* refers to a systematic collection of information translated into behaviour. *Sadvrtta* involves a personal discussion about good conduct and why we choose to behave the way we do.

When we live by the principles of honesty, *sadvritti* (our inner power) develops. *Sadvritti* is personal, social and physical. We should be honest but reserved as we work and live in society harmoniously while facing the complete, unshielded truth when we are alone with our silent selves. Āyurveda describes three sets of specific guidelines for behaviour in society: those for improving physical and mental health, those for proper function in society and those rightful actions that will align us to achieve *moksha*, or ultimate liberation of the soul. Like *sadvrtta*, Āyurvedic principles are grounded in the philosophy of harmony with the universe and cosmos, and are thus often misinterpreted as religion.

Sankhya philosophy espouses that the sense organs, organs of action and body develop from the mind, which creates and controls the body. Hence, the body is ultimately balanced only through the mind. Mere physical treatments are not enough. We must be aware of the mind's three *guna*s or great qualities, called *mahaguna*s. These are *sattva, rajas* and *tamas*. *Sattva* describes balance and harmony, while *rajas* and *tamas* create imbalance. *Rajas* increases agitation and dynamism, and *tamas* increases dullness, heaviness and ignorance. Desire, anger, greed, pride, addiction, fear, worry, jealousy and negative mental urges are due to *rajas* and *tamas,* which also aggravate *vāta*, *pitta* and *kapha*, causing physical disease. *Sadvrtta* increases *sattva*, which restores health, happiness and peace, preventing mental and physical diseases.

While Āyurveda condones the expression of physical urges and encouraged the suppression of psychological urges, modern society often encourages the opposite! Politeness requires that we not allow bodily sounds to emanate from our bodies. Yet, somehow, mental urges that are associated with the seven deadly sins are not forbidden. They fuel capitalist society and only a few of the mental urges are verbally resisted, as few laws prohibit them. Much of society today actually encourages expression of these emotional *vegās*.

Known in Sanskrit as the *mānasika vegās*, or psychological urges, the expression of these *ripu*s (or enemies of the mind) are considered a sign of lack of control over the mind. The Sanskrit terms are *lobha, irsya, dvesa, kama, krodha, mada, moha, matsarya, raga, shoka, bhaya* and *nirlajja*. They have no direct English translation.

Even modern Indian languages have slightly different meanings for the same words. Approximately, they can be attributed to the following:

Ripu	**Meaning**
Lobha	Greed or temptation
Irsya	Envy of another's success/property or jealousy
Dvesa	Aversion to a person, with hostility, hatred or anger that sometimes manifests as fear
Kama	Excess engagement in sensual pleasures, sometimes seen as lust or desire
Krodha	Bitterness that leads to disharmony and anger, rooted in hollowness from insecurity and lack of self-worth
Mada	Excessive expression of ego, also known as *ahankar*
Moha	Uncontrolled desire and over-attachment to sensual pleasures, also expressed as temptation or addiction
Matsarya	Competitiveness, jealousy, which manifest as argumentativeness and prone to disputes rather than observing, remaining calm and quietly determined
Raga	Excessive attachment and passion towards issues in the maya of the material world, sometimes expressed as anger
Shoka	Unbridled grief
Bhaya	Fear not living in the present or being fully aware of one's surroundings
Nirlajja	Shamelessness, due to misunderstanding the context of living in society

Āyurveda also discourages other over-expressions of the mind, body or senses. It discourages the urge to work beyond one's own capacity, advising it will lead to frustrations and interrupted harmony between the mind and body. It discourages wrong thinking, wrong speech and wrong actions, about the self or others. Wrong is defined as anything that goes against the conscience and instinct. If we ignore instinct, we disrupt the cord between body and mind.

Negative emotions, such as fear, worry and jealousy, upset the mind's calm and contribute to interrupting the clean flow between the soul's purpose and the body's work. The urge to use negative speech hurts others and interrupts the innate conditioning of harmony and love that we are born with. The urge to commit wrong that our conscience tells us are not good—such as stealing, robbing and killing—instils disharmony in our mind. All of these urges are considered active poisons that interrupt the highways of positivity and constructive being. Though it sounds philosophical, Āyurveda grounds all mental processes with eventual physical manifestation.

But, how do we cope when we have such emotions spurting forth from our minds? We are often forced to keep them pent up in the Western world, because we are not free to speak our thoughts or act as we feel we must, even when those actions, thoughts and deeds would be positive.

Āyurveda gives three points of counsel: spend time in nature, cultivate close relationships of trust and love, and go inward and reconnect daily—doing construction and repair work on the scaffolding of your mind.

Easier said than done, for a novice these seem near impossible. We hire psychologists and psychotherapists to teach us how to navigate the complicated world of relationships, with others and with self. Āyurveda however, instructs us to anchor our hearts in nature. There are too many fine checks and balances in nature to allow errors, and everything happens for a reason. Therefore, if we observe nature, we can learn how to alter the flows of our thoughts, actions and words so that we can regain harmony and live in peace.

- Negative emotions, such as fear, worry and jealousy, upset the mind's calm, the soul's purpose and the body's work.
- Learn to express physical urges and suppress over-expression of psychological urges.
- To process negative emotions and repair the mind,
  - Spend time in nature
  - Cultivate close relationships of trust and love
  - Go inward and reconnect daily

In most countries, especially in the West, a person exuding body odour will be admonished. At work, the person may be requested to go take a bath, as his/her odour disturbs the peace of those near him. People are encouraged to use deodorants, anti-perspirants, perfumes, body sprays, scented mists, musk oils and perfumed lotions. Smelling nice is part of good grooming.

But in how many places is mental body odour monitored? A person may emit mental odours, such as the stench of anger and a hot temper. No one will request the person to clean his/her mind, mood and mouth. Āyurveda talks about the cleaning of the mind, the mental body bath. This requires attention to the bath, for all the symbols of cleaning that it is.

Besides non-suppressible urges, which are physical actions expressing *vāta* for the function and well-being of the body, and suppressible urges, which are the mental urges of the unevolved and immature mind, there are *vachika dharaniya vegās*—the suppressible urges of verbal expression. These include excessive talking, speaking in extremes, aggressive speech with others, use of harsh words, backbiting, lying and the use of untimely words or irrelevant speech. Mastering control over them provides powerful tools to the mind.

In the *gurukula*, my teacher lectures on the tongue. He posits that control of the tongue is among the most difficult tasks in modern, urban Western society. On one hand, the need to feed our tongue makes us chase food. We become unable to withstand hunger, learning it is normal to become angry when we are hungry. We lose focus on other pursuits as we stuff our faces with things that taste delicious just for a minute. We are slaves to the 'foodie' mentality, unaware that it is simply a marketing tactic. We do not cultivate the teachings of hunger, through *upavasa* (the science of fasting) or through control over *apathya* (food and choices that are not good for us).

On the other hand, the tongue can be dangerous, damaging relationships with hurtful words. Excessive talking prevents people from seeing who we are in our silence. Silence has power in it. To know me when I am silent, when no words are expressed, means to understand me. Speaking in extremes amplifies drama and prevents people from moving forward smoothly. It is commonly used to catch people's attention but also their disdain. Aggressive speech with others is a common tool for control and power. It is often taught in the medical hierarchy as a way to quickly get emergencies under control when saving lives. I learnt it in the emergency rooms during my medical education and was taught to use it when immediate leadership and control is required. Any other use is not judicious and reflects lack of power on the inside.

The use of harsh words is another tool for shocking people; they retreat from the call to battle inviting conflict. Backbiting is the reflection of *matsarya*. Lying is the malalignment from *sanatana*; it decreases one's power. Many will say it is necessary for living in today's society, but it should be remembered that lying is a trade-off between cultivating inner power and averting potential danger or conflict.

The use of untimely words or irrelevant speech dilutes one's inner power by releasing energy into the universe that may not serve any focused purpose. Keeping these concepts in mind develops power and awareness.

If one is truly hunting for power, Āyurveda advises spending part of each day learning about *sadvrtta*. Power originates from the inside, not from wealth, family name, age, fame or forced respect from codified laws of our profession. True power derives from moral strength and spiritual mastery, leading us through life in control of our minds, actions, thoughts and words.

- Cleaning the mind is as important as cleaning the body.
- Control over one's tongue prevents negative energy from being released, encourages better communication and lends control over the appetite.

~ • 27 • ~

Pūja: The Act of Worship

At every morning and night *sandhya* since before I was born, my mother has lit a fire at the altar. She would spend a few moments there, light some kind of candle or oil lamp, some *agarbatti* or incense, and chant a handful of mantras to different sources of power within us, given iconic names to symbolize energies that make them gods.

There are actually three *sandhya*s (meaning joint in Sanskrit) each day: the interfaces between night and day, between day and night and at high noon, when the sun shifts from rising to setting.

At the time of the rising sun, trees switch from making long sugars to using the energy of sunlight to draw carbon from carbon dioxide and hydrogen from water to make precursors of sugar and expel their waste product (oxygen) through leaves. This process is called photosynthesis. From first light until dawn, when the violet and red wavelengths of light penetrate the acute angle of the sky's atmosphere, plants make the most oxygen. During the day, more colours of visible as well as ultraviolet light penetrate, producing less-efficient photosynthesis. At the day's end, plants turn off their photosynthesis machinery and convert sugar precursors from their work all day into storage carbohydrates, building blocks for making leaves, flower buds, roots and fruits. At the *sandhya* of high noon, they get the signal to change their angle ever so slightly, signalled by the sun's posture shifting from rising towards setting.

These three times are worshipped because the junctures represent times of great movement in that zone where the sun is rising or setting. Like a workforce leaving a factory, creating a mass of movement and traffic and noise, there is a subtle mass movement of energy among the trees in unison, shifting between energies of work. This mass movement is a subtle *vāta*, which also exists in the human body as micro-currents and flows of movement in physiology.

As a mass of *vāta* sweeps the earth for hundreds of miles in that time zone, the mind is also subject to that *vāta*, making it prone to sudden changes. If the mind is in chaos, it may not notice the subtle energy change in the trees and plants. But walk through a forest at dawn and the change is more obvious. 'Things are waking up,' people will say. If the mind is stilled during this time of change, it can get swept into that harmonic flow of changing gears that all the plants and animals do in unison and become powerful with the winds of nature. It can also release its chaos, and over many episodes, become conditioned to quickly centre, just as a singer conditioned properly knows how to find his/her own *sa*.

- A few moments to focus on mantras, a light and sweet smell each day at sunrise and sunset pūja create a conditioned mind.

❧

The Sanskrit root *pūj* means to honour, worship, respect, revere and regard. There are two worships of *agni* during pūja: reverence to the fire of the sun and worship of the fire in the firepit, *havana* or candle. Both symbolize the power of transformation for our daily lives. We do pūja daily as a tribute, to partake in the energy of change, with hope for guidance and evolution of our soul.

The great Āyurvedic sage Atreya (Caraka Samhita, Sūtra-sthāna; chapter 8, sloka 28) instructs us to clean our lips, feet and hands, and sprinkle water over the eyes, ears, nose, mouth, heart and head before we sit in order to imbibe energies. Once purified, we offer the fire items that symbolize strength and energy, such as ghee, rice grains, sesame seeds, *khus*, grass and mustard seeds.

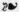

The best time to meditate is after your bath or shower, once you have dried off and gotten dressed. Even if only for a few moments, Āyurveda advocates prayer and meditation just after the body has been cleaned and rinsed with water. Another round of *pranayama*, as described in chapter 19, will quiet the mind and focus the body for some time in *sthira* and *sthana*.

Though meditation is the mental shower after the physical shower, it is not the usual option for most modern, urban in-a-hurry professionals or those living in a house full of people. It should be prioritized however, as a way of cleaning the mind of its odours just as the body is cleaned daily of unwanted dirt and toxins.

- Even if you find only a few moments to meditate, do take time out of your schedule.
- The best time to meditate is after the bath.

❧

At sunset each day, we sit for prayer. Whoever was at the house was welcome. '*Om namo okhondo mandalakarana*' . . . Each and every day, we would be called in from play, from homework and from chores to wash our hands, feet and eyes, light a candle and some incense, recite prayers beginning with the sacred mantra, the Guru Pranam and wish wellness on all our loved ones, especially our sisters. Particularly if we had fought that day, it was both reminder and punishment that siblings were kin and therefore, had to be forgiven before we headed away to another land during sleep. I was proud of my recitations, though I had no idea what the words meant or what language they were in, since they did not sound Bengali. My mother just cascaded through, chanting in her beautiful, strong voice '*Hare Krishna, Hare Krishna*', and we joined in.

Each morning after his bath, Babi insisted I join him in the prayer room. In Princeton, we converted a cedar walk-in closet on the top level of our house. Three walls were covered with our beloved pictures of Krishna, Kali, Durga and Shiva. There were conch shells, *sindhur* in an ancient wooden tantric bowl, fresh flowers and a *narayan shila*, a sacred stone that held quiet forces within.

Anyone that owned or was privileged to be the caretaker of a *narayan shila* had to do proper pūja and maintain their home in a clean, pure way to respect the energies of this god that occupied the stone and the home. Babi had been handed the *shila* on a visit to Haridwar, the sacred city of the confluence of holy men, where the Kumbh Mela happens every twelve years. It is the entry point to the Char Dham, the four main centres of pilgrimage in that region. There, a man had recognized my Babi's unusual energy and had gifted him with this responsibility. My mother was elated. For a Brahmin's wife to worship an actual *shila* means health, wealth and prosperity for her children, possibly because water from its daily bath contains rare trace minerals required for optimal functions of enzymes and the immune system. People come from far and wide to visit our prayer room, giving alms for their children, coaxing their children to approach the altar and praying for focus and strength, usually before an exam or competition.

But for us, the *narayan shila* has become a member of the family. We adjust our schedules to the needs of this energy force. One day, a sceptic Indian physicist and his Nobel Prize-winning colleague visited. They noticed a large pūja was in session for *purnima*. Curious, they watched and then scoffed, engaging my father in a long discussion over the useless icons of religions and how these rocks, following of the cycles of the moon and superstitious worshipping kept India stuck as a Third World country. Forced to defend my family, I quietly retorted that the Third World had ended with the Cold War's destruction of the Second World, and that the First World was filled with plenty of people who believe in saints, holy wafers and the power of blood to turn to wine.

The discussion turned to proving scientific value to these rituals of millions of Indians, many of whom were intelligent professors and scientists themselves. Since subtle energies of electromagnetic fields can be measured by magnetometers, they proposed that my father get a Teslameter or Gaussmeter and measure the opening of the *narayan shila*.

When my mother learnt of this, she vehemently opposed it. 'Why are you violating the energy space of the *shila*?,' she demanded. 'If it is truly strong, it will not mind its field being penetrated,' they countered. She talked about contaminating the energy of a sanctified space and the dangers of interrupting clean environments. She used several analogies of violation: rape, pointing guns and subjecting innocent children to violent sounds, all of which when removed would show that their presence had not been innocuous.

Babi conceded to the scientists, knowing that evidence was the way of the ancients. A Gaussmeter was brought to the lab in our home, and the *narayan shila* was taken there. When the probe was inserted into the hole, the needle flew to the far end past the 1000

Gauss and would not return. Zeiss customer service was called. They asked us if we lived near a nuclear power plant. The instrument was sent for repair, and the experiment continued. Six inches from the *shila*, the field would rise to 10 Gauss. As the probe was brought within a millimetre of the *shila*, there was an exponential rise in the electromagnetic field. The instrument was sent for repairs thrice, each time the probe was inserted, and finally, the experiments were abandoned—to my mother's relief. The scientists disappeared. We later learnt that one had fallen sick for a few months and the other had faced unusual betrayal and financial problems that kept him from visiting. They agreed that later, when things had settled, they would come again to conclude the experiments.

When we told our Indian friends of this adventure, they were quiet. 'Of course there is a force,' the Brahmin men retorted. 'You can feel it when you touch it. You can feel it when your mind is still. That is why we sit near, to imbibe its energy and condition our body with its intensity,' they said. It is why temples are filled with the *shila*s, so that people can go and meditate and do pūja, to increase the power of their minds.

❧

~ • 28 • ~

Choosing Dress

In our bathrooms, we generally had huge mirrors canvassing the entire length of the bathroom, from ceiling to the moulding above the sink. During our free moments, we would drape colourful towels over each other and stand in front of the mirror, modelling our made-up evening gowns, hair turbans and wrap-around skirts, as we tried to coax each other into finishing our bath routines. We would use a dozen towels, as evidence that we had spent sufficient time in cleaning routines in the bathroom. Those long sheets of cotton in different colours, textures and sizes inspired me deeply, showing I could look very different depending on how I draped myself. I began insisting on clothes in particular colours, taking my mother's saris and wrapping them wildly during play.

My maternal grandmother's family in Kashi was connected to one of the famous Benarasi silk mills of the kings. Since childhood, I had seen my mother wearing gorgeous classic saris, with very sparse intricate metallic work and six metres of beauty emanating from solid spun pure silk. Babi's natural choice for most occasions was Benarasi silk, khadi or Bangladeshi cotton. From these fabrics, I learnt about the power of dress.

kāmyaṁ-yaśasyamāyuṣyamalakṣmīghnaṁ-praharṣaṇam|
*śrīmat-pāriṣadaṁ-*śastaṁ-*nirmalāmbaradhāraṇam||95||*

Wearing clean apparel enhances the allure of the body, augments the reputation, increases longevity and prevents penetration of inauspicious nature. It brings pleasure of mind, gives grace, promotes beauty and competence to participate in gatherings with good appearance and confidence, and enhances recognition in society.

Caraka Samhita,
Sūtra-sthāna; chapter 5, sloka 95

During public health training, the history of hygiene teaches that the Greek goddess Hygeia was the personification and epitome of health. Epidemiology explains how Europeans in the 1800s discovered the connection between washing of hands and disease, and why patients died when doctors travelled in the same clothes from patient to patient hurriedly. We learnt about wearing lab coats and sterile fields, the use of sterile gloves and scrubs and the importance of understanding contamination and control of infectious diseases.

However, the first records of hygiene are clearly in the Vedas. From the time of the great sage Atreya and his student Agniveśa, (circa 900 BCE), to the redactor of the knowledge, the acharya Caraka, circa 200 CE, specifics of hygiene documented in detail the rules for diverse societies that lived over that millenium. The concept of *krimi* or microbes is described. They knew dirty clothes can promote illness by keeping the body in contact with harmful factors. They knew the need for bathing regularly to ward off disease. They specifically advise not to wear clothes that have already been worn or to walk on dirty clothes.

Āyurveda counsels us to dress in natural fibres that breathe. Specific cloth is described for specific seasons: cotton for summer in light colours to reflect light; wool in winter to ward off wind and preserve body heat; silk, known as *kauseya*, for protection from rain and wind, but especially in layers for warmth and a single layer for coolness; and linen made from fragments of straw, seeds and fibres, for warding off heat.

Āyurveda also mentions specific ways of dressing for the winter: cotton next to the body, then silk, garments braided with altered wool and silk—called *praveni*—and hides of animals, such as antelopes and sheep. It advises the use of warm, light blankets and rest on bedding covered with *prāvāra* (cotton).

Āyurveda tells us succinctly to dress well. Fine classic weaves have clean lines and please the eye. The colours of the chakras were often used, using dyes made from plants and minerals to instill colours that enhance the desired mood. Gems and metals were also sewn onto clothes, not only for protection from invading knives and possible wounds of war, but also to enhance the body when the metal touched it. Gold was known to enhance immunity, so gold threads were sewn to the borders of saris where they might touch the arms, chest, back and feet. Silver was known to cool inflammation, so silver threads were sewn to the borders of sleeves and necklines. Copper was known to be antiseptic, so copper alloy threads were used for outside protective clothing during war. Gems were sometimes attached with metallic threads for reputed combined effects when touching the body, especially where blouses and scarves touched blood vessel points.

Āyurveda advises choosing colours aligned with *jyotish* and provides a combination of reasons for wearing certain colours on certain days to maximize productivity, usually tailored to a person's forecast. General guidelines also exist.

Day	Colour	Purpose
Monday (Moon day)	White dress and white flowers	To invigorate
Tuesday (Mars day)	Red clothes and red flowers	For success
Wednesday (Mercury day)	Green clothes	To enhance cerebral faculties
Thursday (Jupiter day)	Yellow or off-white clothes	To offer gratitude
Friday (Venus day)	Very light blue or blue-white clothes	To invoke the healing energies of the day
Saturday (Saturn day)	Black clothes and purple flowers	For humility and smooth resolve
Sunday (Sun day)	Pink or maroon clothing, and flowers at home	To enhance relationships

Āyurveda also prescribes not wearing cut cloth in the hot months between April and October. Highly breathable textiles with light weaves were draped as dhoti, *veshti*, lungi, sari, shawl, *shtol* and a loose sarong-type cover. Only after the Muslim and British conquests did women begin to wear cut and tailored blouses with their saris. Cut shirts and trousers helped men and women cope with the mountainous environments of the Himalayas.

❧

One of my patients had a persistent case of skin tags on the neck. She seemed healthy, with good hygiene. Even after multiple cryotherapy surgeries to remove the tags, the problem always returned a few months later, no matter the season. She tried creams, salves and steroid ointments. Since the dermatologist had told her skin tags were benign and the standard safest treatment was simple periodic cryotherapy, her biggest concern was not her health and the underlying cause. It was her inability to comfortably wear bikinis, evening gowns and halter tops. Like most benign skin issues, she had neglected it until it was unsightly.

As is common today, she sought out Āyurveda as a last resort. Āyurveda correlates skin problems with imbalanced *rakta* and *mamsa dhatu*s. *Rakta* is the organ of nourishment that corresponds most closely to the blood and is fed by the gut. Treatment can be delivered through the skin but must pervade the deepest blood. *Mamsa* corresponds to muscle and affects skin as well. Hence, internal cleansing of tissues is vital for cure. She began a course of blood and liver cleansing with herbs such as *manjishtha* and *amalaki* as I created a formulation tailored to her baseline *dosha* constitution, level of digestive fire, lifestyle and *dosha* challenges in her environment.

I also dipped an old pure cotton scarf of hers in a decoction of neem bark powder and let it air-dry in the shade to avoid losing its volatile oils. She was to sleep at night with the scarf wrapped around her neck, wash it after 10 days and re-dip in the neem powder from which she would make a decoction. After two months, she appeared in my clinic, without any skin tags or scars.

Ayurvastra is the science of using clothes medicinally. Āyurveda advocates the embedding of medicinal herbs such as turmeric, neem and tulsi into cotton cloth for wearing against the skin. Transdermal medicinal effects give the person a sustained release of medicine. For many years, a hit item in Arabian countries has been the neem-soaked-and-dried burkhas. These eliminate many of the unsightly skin ailments that people suffer from when they are deprived of sunlight exposure. Other items gaining popularity are cotton scarves or cotton leggings soaked in turmeric. Neem scarves can be used for neck rashes as well as skin tags. Pillow covers soaked in neem can be used for face rashes. Turmeric undershirts can be worn around the house under an old sweatshirt as well. The key to *ayurvastra* is finding good-quality cotton textile that will hold the herb and then release it, dispensing it to the skin gradually when warmed.

- Wear natural fibres, using cotton and linen for summer, wool for winter and silk during the monsoon.
- Clothes and pillow covers dipped in neem and dried can be used to treat skin conditions.
- Use clothes dipped in turmeric and dried too.

~ • 29 • ~

Travel

Ours is a travelling family. Perhaps because my father and mother were outcast from a society that is disdainful towards orphans, high achievers and those who worship truth, they found their own way without their native society. Both were ridiculed and ostracized, and denied due rights of property and position, first by war and then by the mediocre people in their own families and neighbourhoods, who often determine such things through bullying and pulling strings with officials. In the end, both travelled away from their homeland, taking their knowledge and values for living, but venturing forth to adapt them in a new land. It had been the same tradition for generations of women in the family, who emigrated from their homes through weddings to new families.

The current generations of our clan are dispersed around the world, living in seven countries and occasionally holding gatherings for celebrations, weddings, graduations, births and deaths. We have learnt to travel regularly. Even Babi has travelled thousands of miles since the stroke, via advanced disability provisions on airplanes to attend his daughters' graduations, weddings and celebrations. Life in several countries and diverse cultures has accustomed us to journeys and the challenges therein.

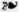

Āyurveda does not care about political and social boundaries. Its laws are based on larger, ancient and earth-sweeping parameters. Where there is disharmony of the flows of wind, there will be problems of *vāta* imbalance, then aggravation, vitiation and finally, derangement. Where the fires of transformation in the body are not harmonious, food and information from the environment will not be properly digested. These will build up as *āma*, undigested residues and *pitta* imbalances. Where there is improper flow and digestion, things will not be stable but either sticky or excessively phlegmy and unable to lubricate or provide the optimal protection and immunity to the body that *kapha* describes. When we travel, we thus put ourselves at greater risks of encounters with the unusual and promote *dosha* imbalance.

Āyurveda advises specifically about travel because it knows that people's routines are altered away from home. Especially now, within hours, travels can alter our time zones, climates, altitudes and hemispheres, as well as food, water and basic staples. These sudden changes unsettle the body's usual expectations, called *satmya*.

Pointing towards epigenomics, Āyurveda discussed the concept of *satmya* as the conditioning of the body in its usual environment. *Satmya* concludes that a person's ideal approach to health and wellness is determined by those foods, climate and behaviour he/she is exposed to during upbringing. Those choices in eating, thinking and breathing create a particular balance that each person maintains inside. According to Āyurveda, This is one of the reasons why the same treatment cannot work successfully for two people with the same disease symptoms. Epigenomic changes to DNA expression occur based on a person's chemical environment, nutritional influences or edible toxins and preservatives that make their way into the DNA and an individual's specific gut microbiome. Āyurveda treats unhealthy epigenomic changes with individualized prescriptions that simply reassert that body's balance of *vāta*, *pitta* and *kapha,* following 'whole-system' effects rather than biochemistry.

When going out into the world, Āyurveda suggests pre-planning. Carry good footwear, an umbrella, covering for the head and body, and a long stick for guiding the path and moving obstacles from the way. Knowing we are prone to *vāta* imbalances inherent to changes in flow of movement when we travel, Āyurveda recommends we lower our *vāta* before departing for journeys by taking time to meditate, be centred and eat food that will not create indigestion.

In my suitcase lives an Āyurvedic emergency kit containing small plastic bags, travel bottles and little glass jam jars filled with cloves, cinnamon, cardamom, *jeera* (cumin seeds), *ajwain*, neem, *guduchi*, ghee, *nasya* oil, mustard oil, sesame oil and *attar*. There is also a small mirror, a toothpick, *anjana* and a small cotton towel for insulation. The cloves and cardamom act as mouth fresheners and can also be added to tea to warm it if the weather suddenly turns cold. Jeera can be combined with warm sesame oil and applied below the navel to relieve unexpected lower abdominal spasms or menstrual cramps.

Ajwain and neem are great emergency medicines for gastroenteritis, nausea or indigestion, especially when suspecting food poisoning. These stimulate the digestive fire and burn out anything that should not be there. Guduchi boosts immunity. Ghee is a moisturizer, dry eye reliever and great for cuts and wounds. It is applied to the eyes at bedtime to balance the *dosha*s and lower *pitta* and *vāta*.

Nasya oil cleans dirt that gets into nostrils and moistens them. Mustard oil is great before baths in cold weather and is rubbed vigorously on the soles of the feet at the first sign of a cold or head stuffiness. Sesame oil is rubbed into the feet before bed to lower *vāta*. *Attar* is an emergency for foul body odour or dirty encounters. *Anjana* is for protecting the eyes from foreign unwanted energies during travel. The small cotton towel is placed over baggage or used as a pillow cover to keep the face protected during sleep while travelling.

Āyurveda reminds us that we cannot learn the lessons that life needs to teach our soul if we stay indoors, isolated from the world. An important element of life is to live yoga off the mat and experience the outer world so that our mind can mature. Until we toil in the troubles of the world, how can we master the challenge of juggling competing priorities, choosing between things we love, or hearing 'no' when we want something? Travel allows us to meet people of other cultures, see lands and landscapes we did not see in our childhood and have a chance to chase our dreams, whatever they may be and however they may have been formed. If we allow ourselves, our children, our spouses, our siblings or our parents to stay inside, for our convenience or for theirs, we are not supporting their growth. We should encourage them to travel, first in their minds, then in the world.

❧

~ • 30 • ~

Profession

As children, we never saw Babi leave home at nine and return at five at the end of the workday, as children on television did. He would sometimes be gone soon after we arose, and sometimes he would sit sipping tea or visiting people when we hurried off to school. Through the decades, there was a pattern. In Santoshpur, Babi held court of a sort. People would come to him throughout the day and night, for advice, assistance, a phone referral or consultation. His job started later in the day and usually involved meetings and the work of a large landowner. He would meet people and only occasionally leave the house. He would spend hours on the local street corner with other men, sipping tea, smoking a pipe and heavily engaged with the conversation of the Bengali mentality. Occasionally, he would take a round of the house, guiding the work that needed to be done.

In Princeton, he was a different man. He held court during dinner parties of Indian families. People would gather to hear his stories, to ask for consultations. An infertility specialist, he would weave fantastic tales and inspire listening couples with the miracles as a storyteller of modern medical technology. Instead of a regular academic job, he built a laboratory downstairs at home, where he spent a majority of his days. It released him from the politics of academia, the corruptions of the biotechnology pharma world and the competitive nature of commercial groups. He had learnt over decades of betrayal that true science was best done when unemployed with a day job. With mental freedom, his work was his play, his life was his work and his companions were his books and his instruments.

Of course, he expected all his daughters to complete higher education. After struggling to ground himself in America so that our careers could advance, there was no question of whether we would attend college, only which college we would attend and which science we would choose. Our brilliance, test scores, negotiation powers and interview skills—both at home and outside in the world—would determine our fate.

Over time, most of my highly qualified friends with integrity have become 'unemployable'. Our minds work too fast to stay anchored to a job. We are too creative to be forced to sit in a box all day. We do not like dishonest agendas. We are our own bosses, writing grants, practising medicine or law, founding non-profit organizations or becoming entrepreneurs to make changes in the world. We are consultants, working on our own schedules. We go where we want, when we want. We earn what is required for our values. We focus on competence, not importance.

bhavati-cātra-vṛttyupāyānniṣēvēta-yē-syurdharmāvirōdhinaḥ |
śamamadhyayanaṁ-caiva sukhamēvaṁ-samaśnutē ||*104*||

Āyurveda suggests that we should choose a path of livelihood that does not clash with the paths of virtue. The path of peace and one that engages a person in his/her studies of interest are preferred, as the mind will be motivated to work. Wealth, virtue and desires can then be attained to lead a fulfilled life.

Caraka Samhita,
Sutra-sthāna; chapter 5, sloka 104

❧

Āyurveda suggests we choose work according to our *prakrti* or baseline *dosha* constitution. It suggests that people with high *kapha* dominance in their *dosha*s will prefer stable jobs with sweet colleagues and comfortable offices. They will tend to forego promotions and challenges to maintain steadiness and stability. People with high *pitta* dominance in their *prakrti* seek careers to change the world; they are ambitious and strong-willed. They like to create challenges at work, making everyone work a little harder because they like to work and because they have a vision to make the company a better place. Those with high *vāta* in their *prakrti* will prefer movement and changes in schedule, location and people. They are ideal salespeople, conference managers or travelling workers.

Statistically, most of us have two *dosha*s that dominate our constitution, though the myriad of combinations and proportions manifest into different *prakrti*s. For each, there are a world of options on what is ideal work. In today's world, dharma's main magical lesson is to love the work you must do if you cannot do the work you love. As you do the work, you will change, learning the lessons your soul needs to learn that are keeping you in that job. Once you master them, the universe will shift you to a new place. If you are true to yourself and prioritize a calm mind so that you can see what is true, what you love will come to you. When we do not remember dharma in that job where we are now, we may become dominated by unhappiness at work. This manifests first as emotions, then thoughts, neurotransmitters, hormones, imbalance and finally, disease.

By *dosha* predominance, the following may be ideal professions:

Mostly *Vāta*	Mostly *Pitta*	Mostly *Kapha*
Sales, marketing, acting, acting, dancing, teaching, writing, photography, designing and so on.	Management, medicine, finance, politics, leadership, law, advocacy and so on.	Administration, nursing, being a homemaker, building, counselling and so on.

Most of today's population lives the day off the mat, working primarily to make money to buy happiness, not spending time with love, the mind unyoked from the body and discontented. Especially now, when there is great mobility in jobs, family status, homes, companies and relationships, there are countless opportunities to manifest your dreams. Āyurveda advises us to live more connected to our hearts, using our profession as our test for assessing what we learnt about yoking the mind and body when we were on the yoga mat. If you can maintain the same calm, connected way of being off the mat, you will have mastered how to manifest true power and the wellspring of true health.

- Practise yoga off the mat even in your professional life
- Be yoked to your heart and mind, even while doing work.

Slow down. In today's world, we are encouraged to move as fast as possible, to multitask, to make lists so we can do more, be more and have more. We learn that time is money. We learn to be human doings and human havings, not human beings. Most companies love workers giving up human needs and working continuously. It may also profit you for some time, but soon it will deplete your strength and vigour. Society tells us this is normal as we age, but when you can no longer work, they replace you without care. Work steadily and replenish yourself regularly so that you can love your work.

We move too fast. Overachieving is rewarded by society. We indulge in the love of doing and the love of creating. When the mind flies, we are free. But if we move too fast, we stumble. The key is to gain prowess in speed-of-light thinking by cultivating the skill of being slow and still, *sthira*. For when we become totally silent, completely still, our *vāta* can re-establish its balance. Only then does our mind re-yoke to our body, senses and soul, and reconnect us to what we really want to do. Once reconnected, we may jump up to speeds that allow completing tasks quickly with fewer errors, more focus and intensity that rips through time without ripping the body.

- Do not overwork yourself. Replenish yourself regularly so that you can love your work.
- Pace yourself. Slow yourself down periodically to nourish and lubricate your gears so you can sustain working fast and hard.

What stopped my father's work was not his brilliance. It was his inability to balance his *dosha*s. His quickened mind and his long working hours made his inspired brain crash into his high expectations and intolerance for deceit. As his work progressed and people tried to suppress his discoveries, his anger surmounted, unresolved from years of neglect in his childhood. Finally, one day, his anger overcame him. I watched Babi's left arm and leg move for the last time, and his speech disappear as the stroke consumed his brain.

Blood pressure rises when the blood vessels and the heart cannot relax and coordinate properly. Called hypertension, high blood pressure is a leading cause of stroke. Years of high pressure on the walls of the blood vessels wear them out, creating patches and rough spots along the arteries and eventually causing a rupture in the ever-flowing rivers. Like a car crash on a highway, the repercussions for the entire road are catastrophic.

Modern medicine labels most blood pressure problems as essential hypertension, confessing that the root cause is not yet known. Āyurveda diagnoses that highly aberrant *vāta* in the blood vessels, combined with small amounts of inflamed *pitta* and some stagnant *kapha* make a troublesome trio and create hypertension. Using this understanding, many of my patients have cured themselves of hypertension. We use a customized approach, analysing how their *prakrti* interposes with their digestive fire and lifestyle choices. Then we make a plan that the person wants to adhere to, rather than a one-sided, hurried prescription. We adjust diet, prescribe mental exercises, promote more physical movement and add *dosha*-balancing herbs. Combination formulas are usually more effective than individual herbs as they prevent unpredictable side effects. The time of day they are taken, known as *bhesajya sevana kaal*, influences how well they are absorbed. The net effect brings down imbalanced *vāta* so that fire in the microscopic channels of the body can rekindle and work optimally. Healthy fire burns out stagnant *kapha* and *āma*. People report that they feel more grounded, more whole and more connected. When they go to work, they handle intensity more maturely, seeing choices not demands.

- Hypertension is a result of highly aberrant *vāta* in the blood vessels, combined with small amounts of inflamed *pitta* and some stagnant *kapha*.
- The time of the day when *dosha*-balancing herbs are taken influence their effectiveness.

❧

~ • 31 • ~

Relationships

When we were younger, even after the loudest arguments between my parents—in which it seemed the house would crumble and the family would break eternally—the next morning my mother would emerge from one of the bedrooms and make a cup of tea for my father, silently asking me to sit aside until she had concluded. Sometimes, Babi would go find my mother and call her to spend daybreak. In those ever-new days, my parents demonstrated the principles of forgiveness, lack of ego and commitment to their relationship. Despite all the disagreements, tortuous issues and never-ending complications of relatives, world events and responsibilities, my parents remained backbones for each other, bound by a silent commitment made at the feet of God one silent April afternoon between two orphaned children trapped in adult bodies.

This puzzled me as a child, because I had learnt from the Mahabharata that truth was the highest ideal. Their arguments certainly reflected their own truths, each of which was argued vociferously. I could not reconcile how such vehement perspectives could melt overnight. But dharma, the principle of living in harmony, both with one's internal energies and external environment, seemed to trump all other ideals.

In this large house now, decades later, with the open boxes calling my parents to conclude chapters of their lives and move forward to a downsized life, I watch my father struggle between his role as her backbone and his desire to continue living indulgently in a house that he can no longer help maintain. After the stroke, he cannot tend to the gardens, grounds, second house or the cars, repairs and lab he has downstairs. My mother cannot manage his growingly frail body, all the stairs in this house and all the falls he has sustained.

Thus, the children have forced the decision to move out of this beloved house, to ease the struggle that the material world has become for Babi, whose soul is trapped in his decaying body. We are all struggling because we love this house and know it intimately. But we also know that being attached will make us mentally unhappy, and that is the root of physical illness. So we are learning to let go.

❧

Āyurveda talks of relationships in the context of a wholesome life. In the thirtieth and last chapter of the Sūtra-sthāna, the great teacher Caraka begins with the purpose of the heart. Then he gets serious, abandoning the poetic rhyme of metre that dominates the book and lapses for twenty slokas into prose format called *gaddi*. He defines the reason why man should even want longevity, defines health and reveals the secrets of *ojas* and how to master resilience and vitality. He then explains the purpose of life, gifting one paragraph on *hita-ahita*, known to all Āyurveda scholars.

tatrā-yuruktaṁ-sva-lakṣaṇatō-yathāvadihaiva-pūrvādhyāyē-ca|
*tatra-*śārīra*-mānasābhyāṁ-rōgābhyāmanabhidrutasya-viśēṣēṇa-*
yauvanavataḥ-samarthānugatabalavīryayaśaḥpauruṣaparākramas
ya-jñāna-vijñānēndriyēndriyārthabalasamudayē-vartamānasya-pa
ramarddhiruciravividhōpabhōgasya-samṛddhasarvārambhasya-
yathēṣṭavicāriṇaḥ-sukhamāyurucyatē|-asukhamatō-viparyayēṇa|-

hitaiṣiṇaḥ-punarbhūtānāṁ-parasvāduparatasya-satyavādinaḥ- śamaparasya-*parīkṣyakāriṇō'pramattasya-trivargaṁ-paras parēṇānupahatamupasēvamānasya-pūjārhasampūjakasya-jñānavijñānōpaśamaśīlasya-vr̥ddhōpasēvinaḥ-suniyatarāgarōṣēr ṣyāmadamānavēgasya-satataṁ-vividhapradānaparasya-tapōjñā napraśamanityasyādhyātmavidastatparasya-lōkamimaṁ-cāmuṁ-cāvēkṣamāṇasya-smr̥timatimatō-hitamāyurucyatē|-ahitamatō-viparyayēṇa||24||*

Those who might live a wholesome life have both earned and been blessed with a multitude of variables. They are not afflicted with physical and mental ailments; they are endowed with youth, enthusiasm, strength, virility, reputation, allure, boldness, knowledge of arts and sciences, good clean perceptive senses, good things to perceive and the ability of the sense organs to interpret them. They have the ability to rightfully gain riches and various articles for enjoying luxury. Those who achieved only what they wisely wanted and moved in the world as they liked, with freedom, have led a happy and wholesome life.

Caraka Samhita,
Sūtra-sthāna; chapter 30, sloka 24

Caraka further elaborates on the mind of those people, saying that if they lead useful lives, they may consider them *hita*, or wholesome.

☙

~ • 32 • ~

Afternoon

After moving to Germany, my parents gradually lost their much-loved routine of napping in the afternoon after a big lunch. Even as they would readily partake in naps when they visited India, when they lived in Cambridge, and then Berkeley, they adapted to the local norm of working each afternoon. In fact, after an early rise and quick tending to the body's morning routine, oiling and bath, and food, they would leave for work and spend the remainder of the day working for others' well-being. When they had jobs, they were at work from 8 a.m. until early evening, and the afternoons were spent in meetings and errands.

Babi now has plenty of time. He moves around the house slowly with his cane and has no particular deadlines, except his daily routines and the occasional calls of nature, his unsuppressible urges. For a few months, my father had taken to watching Oprah and other television programmes regularly. Now, he is on a marathon watching Nova as he becomes proficient with the television's remote control. He will stutter excitedly, sharing the latest scientific discoveries, leaving me to guess what connection he wants to make and what universe he is building in his genius mind, connecting genetics with astronomy, music with botany and chemistry with architecture.

The house is now calling for us to close some of the boxes. No matter how many cartons we finish, seal and send to the garage, when we return to the room, it seems as though the whole room is yet to be packed. Twenty years of life have accumulated, and a month of afternoons cannot clear out what we have collected. This week there will be no siesta.

dharmottarābhirarthyābhih-kathābhistrigunātmabhih |
madhyam-dinasya-gamayodishtśishtasahāyavān || *80*||

In the middle of the day, the period after noon should be spent in the company of like-minded persons, who are also good at heart and helpful in nature. One may also engage oneself in reading stories dealing with the lessons of life, including mostly dharma, some *artha* and a little *kama*.

Astānga Samgraha of Vāgbhata,
Sūtra-sthāna; chapter 3, sloka 80.

After completing the early morning routine, cleansing and nourishing of the senses, the physical bath and the mental bath, the remainder of the day is for our life purpose. Whether with the children, alone, in school, at a job outside home or working in your own shop or company, the day is spent in the outer and not the inner world.

When people want to change their lives, they wonder how a few routines can do it, when most of their hours are spent in a world dominated by other people's priorities. The key to *dinacharya* is to integrate care for the body, mind, senses and soul in the beginning and end of the day, cleaning the senses and kindling the fire, so that whatever enters is cooked to the body's satisfaction to improve the mind and benefit the soul.

Afternoons differ for each person, depending on responsibilities and schedules. But everywhere on the planet, the early afternoon is hotter than the rest of the day and dominated by *pitta*, followed by the period of 3–7 p.m., dominated by *vāta* of the late afternoon. Motivated by the gradually setting sun cooling the skies, plants finish up their day's work of photosynthesis and shift towards their roots, while animals scurry to plan for the night ahead. In cities, people finish work, commute home, plan for the evening or continue with different jobs.

Nature provokes us during these hours of change. Āyurveda advises that we take advantage of the provocation, by smoothing any aberrant flows in our life. This is the time to smooth out tasks yet undone. It is time to ride the wave of movement by getting exercise, a bike ride, a yoga class, a walk in the park or a golf game. Many creative companies schedule brainstorming sessions for this time, unknowingly but instinctively aligning with the etheric highways we tend to travel during these hours. Creative writing, painting and late-afternoon concerts take advantage of this wave of movement as well.

- Use the period of 3–7 p.m. to resolve all work for the day, indulge in hobbies and creative activities or get in some exercise.

In tropical countries throughout the world, napping is the norm for afternoons. It is *satmya,* conditioned normal behaviour for people who are accustomed to the routine of their hot climate. Afternoon temperatures year-round do not permit a golf game, farm work, exercise or time in nature. The only hope to survive the heat accumulating in the air is to retreat into rest and stillness.

For healthy, young and strong people, Āyurveda does not encourage long afternoon napping. It encourages stillness, rest, meditation, reading or *riyaaz* (practice time for music, study and small projects sitting in the sun of winter or shade of summer). If one must nap, Āyurveda advises it be done sitting or leaning, but never reclining fully to allow the head to be horizontally placed. Over time, napping increases *kapha* and is especially discouraged for overweight and diabetic persons, though their urge to doze may be highest because their digestive fire is low. Young children, the elderly, pregnant women, the sickly and the infirmed are permitted to rest and should allow the *vāta* hours to bring stability and calm to them.

- When the afternoons are extremely hot, healthy and young people should spend time in stillness, rest, meditation, reading, practice or on small projects.
- Long naps should be avoided, especially by overweight and diabetic people.
- Young children, the elderly, pregnant women, the sickly and the infirm may rest during these *vāta* hours to imbibe stability and calm.

❧

Part V: Nutrition

As I begin to pack the kitchen of my parents' home, the cupboard of spices—now stained yellow from decades of Indian cooking—is a formidable challenge. A hundred glass jars fill the cupboard, recalcitrant to being packed into boxes easily. The most silent refusal comes from the kitchen *dabba,* the firestick for most of the food consumed by this family for the past twenty years and the centre of this kitchen's family traditions. The spices in the round *dabba* sit in seven inner small bowls with one lid—mustard, *jeera, kalonji, ajwain,* turmeric, *panchparan* and fennel. What is chosen for each bowl reflects each kitchen's slightly different culture, but all Indians know that these spices are *deepana;* they increase the digestive fire. The spices reflect the depth of wisdom among ancestors of the clan who raised those who now cook there. Their judicious use reflects the love of the chef for those he/she feeds and the wealth that arises from having healthy, happy lives that can only happen with healthy bodies and focused, ignited minds. Ultimately, the power of the household lies in this *dabba.*

❧

Part V:
Nutrition

~ • 33 • ~

Food

The game of Āyurveda is actually simple: it is a game of fire. Routines of the day and season are planned around the fire of the sun. Choices of food, exercise and work are planned around the fire of the body. By understanding *dosha*s, we can predict how our fire will react to our choices on any day. If we feed our fire correctly, we will digest all we need to be healthy.

Different rituals exist for different climates from different classical texts, telling us what and when to eat. The chemistry of each food, how it is grown, collected and prepared is detailed, advising us how to influence our *dosha*s with our foods. Āyurveda reminds us that while each person is unique, there are basic unchanging guidelines that depend on the condition of fire in the body.

❧

Āyurveda says there is no bad food, only food that is good for kindling and supporting the *agni*. I prescribe two rules: 1) eat freshly prepared food; 2) know when the food was last living and connected to the earth. If you cannot pinpoint the time it was last living as a plant or animal, do not eat it. It is not food. It is dead chemical stuff and will not be assimilated into the live, living body as easily. These two rules eliminate a lot of issues as people find themselves learning how to use stoves, eating better-quality food and eating what their bodies really want.

These two rules about food will hold you in good stead:

- Eat freshly prepared food
- Avoid food that is full of preservatives and extensively processed.

One evening, I was invited to dinner by one of my dear friends, a young Āyurvedic physician. As he came down to receive me, he led me to the market where we purchased some fresh vegetables before we climbed to his fifth-floor apartment. As I assisted unpacking, I noticed he had no refrigerator. My judging mind began to calculate why he did not have the time, money or effort to furnish his kitchen. He had a full range of spices, utensils and pans, and was financially comfortable.

Finally, I asked him. He looked at me, amused, and answered that he was not so poor that he had to eat dead food and could afford the time and energy to prepare meals fresh three times daily. He had sufficient knowledge about food storage and which food not to consume. He explained that people who did not have true wealth were those lacking understanding about food preparation, storing precooked food, killing food with cold and underestimating the importance of fire. Poor people have refrigerators or eat outside food because they cannot afford fresh home-cooked food, he quipped, reminding me of his small village.

Over six months, he showed me how to store milk overnight, how to keep leftover rice safely for use in the morning and how to keep vegetables in the house without bugs or rodents getting to them. He used a pack of neem leaves hanging near the vegetables, whose volatile oils kept predators away. He used cool water to store the rice, rinsing it out in the morning and recooking it for a fresh taste. He kept milk freshly boiled in an iron wok, with a lid over it, and then re-boiled it in the morning for tea. My Westernized ideas about food preservation were transformed.

It is good to stay away from leftover food. While the modern lifestyle counsellor will show you recipes to make on Sunday and eat for a week, taking a portion each night out of the freezer and into the microwave, Āyurveda advocates fresh food to feed a live, fresh body. Despite the convenience and saved time, the investment made by cooking fresh food is in the interest of your health. Only those who cook fresh meals from raw fresh ingredients can appreciate the value of this true wealth.

❧

Part VI: *Ratricharya*: Routines for the Night

Each of these last nights I am in this house, helping to pack and conclude my parents' life in it, I am filled with sentiment. My father can feel it. He has always simultaneously praised and admonished my strong emotional and metaphysical nature. I do not live in one world; I live in a timeless present.

He calls me to him just after the *sandhya* sunset prayer, the boundary between a day and its evening. When we were younger, he would call me to sit and talk for an hour until the news, dinner or a phone call interrupted our session. Now, with his stroke-induced silence, he motions to me to sit next to him as he pulls out an old photo album.

Over the next hour, he opens to different pages and slowly utters names, locations and events, with a memory so sharp that its edge cuts resentment into my whole being that all-knowing neurologists had declared his brain unrepairable and not worth physical therapy five years earlier. He points out chapters of his life, his research career, people who journeyed with him through triumphs and tribulations and those who were called his family, mostly who took from him.

Evenings are periods meant for recounting the day, in gratitude for what we have seen and learnt. It is a time to be with family and relax after the strong, intense energies of the day have blown circumstances into our lives. As the boxes multiply and occupy most corners of these bare-walled twenty-five rooms, we are reminded that this is one of our last evenings in this house. But it is an evening when my father is still with me, and I am grateful that every evening in this beloved house will have been one with him in it. I know that there will be those ahead without him.

Part VI:

Ratricharya: Routines for the Night

~ • 34 • ~

The Evening and Dinner

Throughout our childhood and early adulthood, we were not permitted to speak at the dinner table. For many years, I thought it was because girls should be seen and not heard. We would spend the time passing non-verbal signals to each other and passing things surreptitiously under the table.

We learnt early that Brahmins do not talk during meals because we should spend that time focused on gratitude and how food becomes our bodies, at which point we would giggle at knarled carrots or fat potatoes and point to each other. Despite watching the adults talk while eating, we were instructed to stay quiet because air would get into our bellies with the food. We learnt that quiet eating meant good digestion and more calm tummies at night. My mother was conveying what she had learnt, not knowing it was cultural Āyurveda. For generations, her family lived Āyurveda without calling it Āyurveda, because it had been outlawed as a medical system. All that could safely be preserved by the subjugated Indian people was Āyurveda as a series of cultural beliefs.

Occasionally, my mother would turn from her conversation with my father to us and ask if we wanted second helpings. Otherwise, the entire dinner conversation consisted of my father's conversations about his research on sperm, their count, their motility, their zeta potentials and how their chromosomes stained. We learnt about the biochemistry of seminal fluid, which my father had replicated and patented, and we learnt about the characters and personalities in science that interfaced with my father at the Institute for Advanced Study or Princeton University or one of the other institutes of higher learning where he travelled.

These conversations were usually followed by commands for us to help with kitchen chores and then turn to our homework. But our evenings were often spent rushing between bedrooms, visiting different sisters, sharing stories of the day and news on common friends, showing acquired gadgets and tools from school and planning the next day. The evenings were never lonely unless we sat isolated and did our homework. Those were planned carefully for nights when visitors would come, so that we could show them how studious we were.

My father's friend came to visit from Haridwar one evening. As we prepared for dinner, we asked his preferences, trying to ensure that he was tended to well. He politely declined, saying that he never ate dinner. It was the first time I had heard of this in a person who was not sick. Three square meals was the prescription we had always heard.

He sat down with us and shared some yoga shāstra. His *sādhana*, an act of sacrifice with the purpose of focusing the mind, for the past twenty years had been to not have dinner. I considered his plight: no dessert, no TV dinners and no evening appetizers. He said, *teen bhojan rogi, do bhojan bhogi, ek bhojan yogi*. 'Roughly translated', he explained, 'three meals a day creates a patient; two meals a day creates a sufferer; one meal a day creates a yogi, or person connected with their soul and in control of their body's functions.' Until that time, I had thought that everyone enjoyed dinner unless they were ill or punished.

Over time, I began to watch for dinner habits wherever I went. I found that traditional cultures ate early, before six in the evening, often to avoid eating in the dark. Many farm cultures involved eating the largest meal at 4 p.m., just as the sun was setting, and ate breakfast early before heading to the fields. Most cultures in pre-industrial times planned meals and preparation around the availability of sunlight. As my parents got older, I saw them shift to earlier meals, using the evening gatherings for food-free music, socializing and maybe a light cup of tea, milk or an occasional dessert. The kitchen was basically closed by 7.30 p.m. This, of course, was very inconvenient for guests. However, my mother remained flexible for them, preparing for and serving them jovially, but firm that her family would not partake with the guests, as we had finished our meals.

Living with a royal tribal family in west Africa, I found that the patriarch and senior mothers would eat alone. This stemmed from other concerns. The patriarch did not want people to watch him eat, lest they sent negative energies into his food, commented on his food, changed his mood or distracted him mentally from his connection with his meal. In addition, only two of the seven wives of the house were permitted to prepare his plate. Over time, I began to notice that many elder wise men throughout the world also eat alone, serving and tending to any guests, and then sitting quietly in their own clean environment with time and energy to eat quietly as a meditative exercise, especially if they were eating only one meal per day.

❧

In industrialized cultures, where the schedule often revolves around the daily office or factory workday, a family generally uses the dinner meal as a time for gathering, therefore making more elaborate preparations for dinner. Unfortunately, this results in the dinner meal being the heaviest and often the most unhealthy meal of the day. After-dinner walks have been replaced by shifting to the TV room, if the family did not already have TV as the main dinner companion. The habits of dinner have unwittingly predisposed many to the lifestyle diseases now plaguing society.

After one of my Āyurveda teachers broke his ankle in the US and in the hospital for an extended period, he was nurtured by friends until he could travel. A family of modernized doctors and professionals, they had a typical Western, urban lifestyle. But their hospitality was so warm that he simply adjusted to their schedules for the months he was convalescing.

When he returned home, he began to reinstitute the principles of Āyurveda. He did not suddenly shift, as the body had adjusted to the Western lifestyle for a season. Slowly, he began to eat dinner 15 minutes earlier every few nights, shifting his late-night hunger back to his healthy earlier dinner time. In the beginning, he was not at all hungry for dinner until 9.30 p.m., but slowly, over a couple of weeks of eating slightly lighter lunches, he found his hunger returning around sunset.

His evening meal became light again. He never mixed grains, choosing rice, wheat or millet. If he chose roti, he would not eat rice. He avoided preparations that mixed cow milk with vegetables. He avoided onion and garlic, as their *katu vipaka* (pungency), would heat up the body. Naturally a non-meat-eater, he added more fresh pulpy vegetables to his lunch so that his desire for heavier textures would be met. He added cumin, turmeric and digestive spices to his food to augment his digestive fire and promote forward flow of food through the system, known as *vāta anulomana*. He stopped eating beans and cauliflower at night, as they cause gas and tend to make the night less calm.

After lunch, he returned to his one tablespoon of homemade yoghurt; no commercial versions. Some days, he would have chhaas, yoghurt diluted in water with five spices, to improve digestion and the flow of *agni*. He never had yoghurt with fruit or other dairy products. Because yoghurt is *abhishyendi*, or channel-clogging, he made sure not to have it early in the morning or late at night, focusing on having it only half an hour after lunch when his *agni* was high enough to digest its goodness before it clogged channels.

He also slowly removed dessert, which had become a mandatory part of his hosts' mealtime. As they sipped brandy, he was given something rich and sweet to indulge him; sometimes cakes, sometimes ice cream and sometimes fruits. Fruits are *sattvic* foods, to be eaten separately when the stomach is empty. For best effect, Āyurveda suggests they not be combined with anything else. Eating fruit at the end of a meal throws it into the cauldron of food being digested, promoting indigestible portions. He shifted his fruit intake to late afternoon and stopped mixing citrus fruits with other fruits.

Simplifying his food types and eating one course at a time, he realigned his food order, preparation and composition with Āyurvedic medicinal recommendations, especially because he had recently been ill. He chose fresh vegetables every day, based on his morning appetite, making access to a fresh farmer's market a priority. He chose luscious food and good recipes to promote his anticipation for specific food to release specific digestive enzymes that are released to intensify digestion of that food. He cooked each vegetable according to traditional preparations and combinations, only with its allocated spices. He never ate leftovers and never used pre-made sauces, which generally contain preservatives or previously ground spices that lose their volatile oils days after they are ground.

We have three chances each day to medicate ourselves: breakfast, lunch and dinner. We have three chances each day to poison ourselves and our efforts towards health: breakfast, lunch and dinner. The summation of our decisions around our meals can either undo or augment our efforts using medications, herbs, health regimens and habits. Experienced clinicians of Āyurveda detailed guidelines, describing a science oriented around digestive fire, rhythms of the day and the nature and unctuousness of the body. These guidelines discuss the concept of *viruddha ahara* or incompatible food combinations that challenge the optimal state of the body.

Incompatible Food Combinations	
Milk	Fish
	Meat
	Sour substances
	Salt
	Fruits
	Peas
	Leafy vegetables
Yoghurt	Ghee
	Fruits, especially bananas
Fruits	Vegetables

Most traditional Indian recipes never use these *viruddha* combinations. Only more recent dishes, usually influenced by European or Persian cultures, introduced these combinations to Indian cuisine. According to Āyurveda, these have opposite *viryas*, or thermal potency—a concept studied in modern chemistry around the energy and heat locked in a place or compound. Therefore, they confuse the fire of the body, just as adding hot oil and ice would, and imbalance it.

In a few weeks, losing the burden of disease that heavy dinner creates, my teacher began feeling light again. He then began to walk and exercise his middle body, working mobility back into his spine, his midriff and his hips. He increased his *pranayama* routine before meals to increase his *agni* and monitored his fire, appetite, cravings, bowel movements, sleep cycle, fatigue level and mood.

When his *agni* was back to normal, his glow returned, not only due to his physical health, but also because his self-confidence had grown. He had proven his ability to take himself through a trauma, hospitalization and a disoriented environment in a fast-paced location back to the optimal environment for his body. This re-found resilience was his evidence.

The end of the day is for winding down and *sneha*—tenderness, love and softness. The evening's *kapha* hours, 7–11 p.m., induce slowness as well as grounding. During this time, Āyurveda recommends using the natural tendencies of the *kapha* times of day, when the energies are prone to cold, moisture, heaviness, being grounded, stillness and softness. One can summarize the day to ground its accomplishments, planning for the next day. Spend time with loved ones and laughter to increase heart energy and ground relationships. Sit in warmth as the day's heat is dissipating. Read to share stories, knowledge and depth. Soak food or preparations for the night.

In today's world however, the reality is that people living in cities often work late into the evening. Rather than winding down, they move into a second shift, still commuting and travelling, or preoccupied with work from the day and not ready to conclude. Āyurveda allows the reality of this on some occasions but treats it like a fulcrum. Too much time in movement increases *vāta* or pushing through intense *pitta* activities, especially during *kapha* hours, separates a person from the flows of nature, creating an environment prone to imbalances that may eventually lead to disease.

If one eats supper or dinner, it should be in the earlier part of the evening, lighter than the midday meal and easy to digest. If the body and mind has to spend the following hours digesting food, it cannot focus on the clean-up of the body and the digestion of food that has come into the mind. Thoughts and mental activities of the day must be reconciled in the night, and this can only happen if the body is not busy focusing on the gut. Therefore, Āyurveda says that we will resolve our mental anguishes and increase our intellectual development best if we eat a light dinner and spend part of the evening engaged in activities of love and light.

- Use the evening to wind down the day.
- Summarize and reconcile the events of the day and plan for the next day.
- Spend time with loved ones and in joy.
- Sit in warmth as the day's heat is dissipating.
- Read to share stories, knowledge and depth.
- Soak food or preparations for the night.
- Dinner should be in the earlier part of the evening, lighter than the midday meal and easy to digest.

~ • 35 • ~

Effects of Nature's Seasons: *Rtucharya*

Every few months, my mother would sweep through our closets, bathrooms and kitchen, switching to different toothpastes and oils, and taking out sweaters or putting them away to pull out spring clothes. Grains, oils and spices would be shifted, hot spices for summer pushed to the back of the cupboard in their glass jars and cooling spices, coconut oil and puffed rice shifted to the front.

She would change the newspaper linings on each shelf, in the kitchen cupboards, the pantry and all the closets of the bedrooms and bathroom. 'Cleanliness is next to godliness', she would say. Of course, she would also get us involved. On the weekends, as she would serve breakfast, she would announce our group cleaning activity for the day. Working together, we would chat and clean, making it fun, learning how to divide labour and to compromise between preferences, egos and ideas.

Headstrong, one of us would insist on a particular cleaning plan and quarrel until a debate ensued on the best way to accomplish the task. My mother would challenge us to hold our stand with logic.

'Which comes first, a newspaper to wipe grime or a sponge to apply water? Is cumin a warm weather spice or a cold weather spice? Can we use this object in the summer or only in the winter?' My mother would resolve each debate, teaching why she cleaned in the order she did and why she was shifting things for the seasons.

Each season has a flavour that is based on its energy and the energy's *guna*s. Āyurveda describes ten parameters to describe physical objects. The three dominant ones are temperature, digestibility and unctuousness. *Virya* (temperature) refers to the ability of a given substance to make the body hot or cold. If the body is seen as a container, any object put into that container can make the container hotter (*ushna*), colder (*sheeta*) or leave it unchanged. When we choose foods that have an inherent cooling nature, called *sheeta-virya* in Āyurveda, the food makes our body cooler. Examples are melons, coriander seeds, rock sugar, milk and coconut oil.

Digestibility refers to the body's ability to digest something easily. This can refer to food, thoughts, medicines or words. If something is easy to digest, it is called *laghu*. If it is difficult to digest, it is *guru*, which also means heavy or carrying weight. The term is often limited to a common reference to people who are venerable teachers, but the actual root in Sanskrit refers to moving (*ru*) out of the darkness (*gu*). When we digest information and become clear, we move out of darkness. When we eat something heavy, it takes time and energy to digest and produce energy from it, where energy is light.

Unctuousness (*snigdha*) refers to the quality of being oily and somewhat adherent and sticky, but still smooth. It is the opposite of dry and rough, known as *ruksa* in Sanskrit. When something is very dry, it is difficult to digest. When it is clean-and-fresh oily, it is easier for the body to assimilate it because it is itself oily. Compare old oil with new oil and smell the difference. One is sticky; the other flows uniformly. These qualities relate to the body and the seasons.

The heavy *kapha* season of clouds and snow promotes thick, heavy stickiness. The body counters this by increasing its internal fire to cope with the cold. If the fire is good, it will prefer clean, sharp foods that cut through the heavy cloudiness of the season. As the *kapha* season gives way to the warmth of the *pitta* season, the air turns somewhat hot, windy and acidic. The body responds by decreasing its internal fire and craving colder, sweeter food that neutralizes the acid and the heat. As the hot season folds into a cooler windy season, the lightness of *vāta* with its cold, dry, rough and mobile nature brings chills and movement into the body. The body copes by craving warm and watery food, heavy sweet vegetables, and oils and seeds. Thus, as the seasons roll through their cycles, so must we shift to adjust to the associated *guna*s.

My mother is ritually connected to her pūjas, which revolve around the lunar cycles. In addition to daily pūjas for the *narayan shila*, she does Lakshmi pūja every Thursday. There are also pūjas on the eleventh day of the lunar cycle, called *ekadashi* and a *purnima* pūja with a Satyanarayan pūja on the full moon. I am a bit disturbed by the ritualistic nature of all these pūjas, so I ask why a public health worker married to a logical scientist is doing all these pūjas.

She is very clear our tides are ruled by the moon, the way that the ocean tides are ruled by the moon. We, like the tides, experience waves of movement through our water. These are influenced by the moon. It is difficult to believe in these analogies until we compare with nature. In our own bodies, we can see a mechanism ruled by the lunar movement: our menstrual cycle.

Āyurveda tells us of the benefits of the moon. Not only is its light *pitta*-pacifying, but it is also a magical light, in which the body cools and becomes more soft and emotional. The ultimate treatments for *pitta* disorders, in which inflammation plays a heavy role, is to take a silver cup filled with milk, add a rose petal and place it in the moonlight on a full moon night so that you can see the moon's reflection in the milk. This milk is then given to the *pitta*-aggravated person as an elixir. Silver, milk, rose and moonlight have a cooling effect.

Chemically, the light of the moon is of a different character than the photons of the sun. Photons from the sun that penetrate from long angles have less ultraviolet light, such as at sunrise and sunset. Similarly, the light that bounces off the moon and reaches the earth is also changed because these photons are first absorbed by rocks on the moon and then reflected almost identically, except that the wavelength is slightly longer. The overall effect we perceive is colour change and change. Āyurveda interpreted that these lights both transform the human body; sunlight heats up the body and increases *pitta*, while moonlight cools the body and decreases *pitta* and *vāta*. Physicists studying the moon now confirm that the way light reflects during the full moon differs from that during other moon phases, decreasing its reflection by a power of ten. With no atmosphere or wind, the moon conveys stillness and calm.

> ❧ To remedy *pitta* disorders, usually marked by inflammation, drink milk with a rose petal from a silver cup kept in moonlight.

Āyurveda texts describe changes needed each season, outlining cyclical increases in *dosha*s and the tendencies for imbalance and disease, advising how to counter these natural undulations. For example, as the intensity of cold increases during extreme winter, known as *sisira rtu*, dryness increases, depleting the body's reserve and natural oils. For this, Āyurveda advises daily head and body oil massages and then sitting in the midday heat of the sun. It recommends meat soups, ghee, hot beverages with jaggery and molasses, rice flour, milk products and sesame oil, all rich food with plenty of inherent fats and oil to replenish the body. It advises warm, sensuous embraces and lovemaking after anointment with perfumed musks and fragrances.

Āyurveda then cautions that *kapha* that has increased and accumulated during the extreme winter will begin to liquefy when the sun begins to move back towards the north, called *uttarayana.* This will weaken the digestive fire in the body and promote many *kapha* diseases. Many *kapha*-pacifying and liquefying protocols are thus prescribed for *vasanta rtu*, early spring. These include *nasya*, light diets with warm, watery soups and light, dry preparations, use of *udvartana* before a bath and full engagement in sports and exercises. During this season, old barley and wheat are recommended, alongside grilled preparations of meat that have melted away the fat, and honey with its scraping nature. Specific matured herbal medicinal wines called *asavam* and *aristam* are to be sipped by lovers. Midday is to be spent with friends and lovers, walking in the sunlight and working on cheerful projects. Sleep in the daytime in discouraged, as is sweet, heavy, oily, sour and salty food.

As the sunrays become stronger, the body feels more and more wrung out, with the constant heat of *grisma rtu*, the summer. This time weakens the *kapha* of the body day by day and strengthens the *vāta* and movement. The mind will be quicker, but the lubrication of the body—especially the joints—will be drier. Therefore, one should stay away from direct contact with the sun, strenuous exercise during the day, and salty, sour, acidic, pungent and spicy food. Āyurveda recommends eating sweet fruits; light and oily preparations, such as salads; liquid preparations such as chhaas and light soups; and cooling food such as cucumbers, melons, apples, grapes, most green vegetables, old rice, rock sugar and light milk preparations. It advocates daily baths in cool water and walking in the moonlight.

If one lives according to the seasons, evenings also vary according to the light, heat and flavours in nature and what Āyurveda recommends. In the modern day, temperature variations are largely ignored by us, as we have heated and air-conditioned homes and move from cars into garages into offices and malls and back to home. Modern life has separated us from the natural cycles that challenge our *dosha*s to shift and rebalance, and strengthen our bodies and minds. To re-engage with that cycle of nature, take walks daily according to the season, exercise and switch food to be in tune with the local environment.

- Align your schedules with the seasons through exercise and diet.

During winter, add these to your routine:

- Daily head and body oil massages when healthy, with time for absorbing some midday heat of the sun
- Meat soups, ghee, hot beverages with jaggery and molasses, rice flour, milk products and sesame oil
- Warm, sensuous embraces and lovemaking after anointment with perfumed musks and fragrances

Adopt these into your routine in early spring:

- *Nasya*
- Lighter diets with warm, watery soups and light, dry preparations

- Use of *udvartana* before a bath
- Full engagement in sports and exercises
- Old barley and wheat, alongside grilled preparations of meat,
- Honey, with its astringent, grounding, drying nature
- Matured herbal medicinal wines called *asavam* and *aristam*
- Midday with friends and lovers, walking in the sunlight and working on cheerful projects
- No sleep in the daytime if healthy
- Avoidance of sweet, heavy, oily, sour and salty food

In the summer, use these guidelines:

- Avoid direct contact with the sun once it ascends beyond dawn.
- Minimize strenuous exercise during midday.
- Reduce salty, sour, acidic, pungent and spicy food.
- Eat sweet fruits; light and oily preparations, such as salads; liquid preparations such as chhaas and light soups; and cooling foods such as cucumbers, melons, apples, grapes, most green vegetables, old rice, rock sugar and light milk preparations.
- Bathe daily with cool water, soaking the scalp.
- Walk in the full moonlight.

~ • 36 • ~

Alcohol and Smoking

For many years of my life unbeknownst to me, my sister and I were lushes—slang for women who drink too much alcohol. We tease my mother about her hand in this and dissolve into laughter as she tries to defend herself.

The truth is that when we first arrived in America, it was very cold and we were very irritable at night. We were also very skinny. My mother was at her wit's end on how to nourish us and get some fat on our bones, until a kind neighbour recommended a large smoky bottle and suggested my mother give us some in a tall glass of warm milk as a 'toddy'.

Not understanding enough English to taste first, she would mix a generous portion of this toddy, Rémy Martin with warm milk. My sister and I would sip our tall glasses happily, complete with milk moustaches, and with the sweet bitter taste of toddy in our mouths, we would soon fall asleep. This pleased my mother, so she insisted my father bring the same large bottle home for the next several years until we fattened up enough to resist illness in the new land.

❧

saumanasyakrto-hrddhānvayasyauh-sahitah-pibet |
nirgadānāsavārishtasīdhumāddhīkmādhavān ||22||

One should enjoy drinks of *āsavas* and *aristas*, fermented infusions and decoctions that generate alcohols within, using herbs tended with sugarcane, grapes and honey, that are delightful and delicious—aged for maturity—and mix them with the juice of mango fruit; these should be drunk with friends, flavoured by the sip of the lover, presented with charm and the gracious scent of her body and the grace of her beautiful eyes, to bring satisfaction both to the mind and heart. Water boiled with ginger or *musta* or mixed with honey can also be used by those who should not consume alcohol.

Ashtanga Hrdayam,
Sutra-sthāna; chapter 3, sloka 22

Caraka redacts thirty-five slokas of Agniveśa's wisdom (Caraka Samhita Sūtra-sthāna; chapter 5, sloka 20–55) discussing the details of smoking and providing recipes, size, shape and method to light a medicinal cigar. He prescribes it for the release of excess *kapha* from the head and discusses advantages of smoking *kapha*-reducing herbs. A detailed schedule of the eight times of day when smoking can improve health has been outlined. He delves into treating complications that may arise, discusses contra-indications and disadvantages of smoking and the methods for inhalation and exhalation. Details even include the size and shape of the smoking pipe and how to smoke properly to avoid both excess and medicinal insufficiency.

When we make our own cigars under the guidance of an Āyurvedic physician who knows how to prepare and create the experience of healthy smoking, we can enjoy a smoke without fear. These recipes are not haphazard. They were written and tested in the days of Atreya, circa 900 BCE, used and handed down over time via oral rote and palm leaf, and finally collected around 200 CE by Caraka, who culled, vetted and compiled the knowledge of his forefathers' collections into a compendium, today called his Samhita. The theory and practice of all prescriptions, including smoking, had to meet the definition of medicine: to heal and not harm.

In today's society, smoking is equated with tobacco, and little is revealed about manufacture of modern cigars and cigarettes with excess nicotine, chlorine-bleached paper and synthetic chemicals, submerging their process in the secrecy of patents and profits. Companies use the nefarious process of using thousands of people for production, so that no individual can be blamed for its deleterious effects. In effect, smoking has become an addiction and is no longer the medicinal use of smoke to reach the inner caverns of the sinuses and cavities of the head.

❧

People are often misled to believe that Āyurveda forbids alcohol, smoking and indulgences of the body. Contrary to popular belief, Āyurveda states that there is a time and place for everything.

Not everyone is suited to all activities and intakes. Alcohol is best consumed when the astringency, sharp taste and effects are good for the body: in the dead of winter when *kapha* begins to build up and at the end of a long day, in the evening, during *kapha* hours. It is not to be consumed in excess, as with any medicine. In the windy months and heat of summer, it is strictly forbidden.

When followed according to the parameters of what is good for the body, Āyurveda lets one enjoy the senses without being trapped by them.

- Alcohol is best consumed in the dead of winter and at the end of a long day.
- Do not consume it in excess, as with any medicine.
- Do not drink hard alcohol in the windy months or heat of summer.

~ • 37 • ~

Raticharya: Sex and Intimacy

My sister was born after my mother's tubal ligation operation. My mother laughs when she narrates the tragic story of medical failure, because my sister is the best thing that happened to both our lives. My father had refused to take my mother to a doctor in the US, convinced she was crazy to feel she was pregnant. Finally, he conceded after four months, worried that she may have cancer in her growing belly.

That doctor recommended my mother abort the unwanted child, a remnant of the eugenics movement that had spread through the Midwest in the 1930s, legalized by chapters of the American Medical Association in two states, making abortion and involuntary sterilization on coloured people legal. My mother walked away, stating that this child especially was God's will. The chance of pregnancy after tubal ligation is under one in hundred.

The little baby that came out was very red, very small and very, very lovable. She instantly became the baby of the family and remained my father's favourite even after younger cousins were born. She has an innate survival instinct, an ability to judge lucidly between difficult perspectives and an uncanny advocacy for the underdog. Years later, she specialized in three subjects together, graduating with honours from an Ivy League school and then law school. She now manages the legal issues surrounding the sale of this big house, the property, the trust and the wills.

It was only years after college that I realized why women have tubal ligation done. I had learnt it as a technical procedure in family planning, never considering the relationship aspect of it. In fact, though sex was all around us, as children of a spermatologist, we never really knew what sex meant.

On Oprah's talk show, there is a long week of 'sex special' episodes. Only in the fourth segment on sex basics, 47 minutes into the hour-long episode, does the word 'intimacy' emerge. The real issue around sex is intimacy, baring the soul, mind and body, indulging in the senses and surrendering to the chemical attraction between two beings. People are afraid to engage in true intimacy, which requires both time to develop, a commitment to self-development and maturity in managing one's own desires and needs while allowing vulnerability and at once managing those of one's partner.

Today's society is quick to admit that sex sells. Campaigns optimize subliminal advertising, setting up sexual images and shapes around products based on raw instinct. They appeal to our cravings to stimulate our senses, loneliness, insecurity and desire to be wanted. They exploit our need to be loved.

But watch people with charisma. The real power of sex appeal is that one exudes the ability to engage in intimacy. Their arms are ready to hold another person. They want to engage, as reflected in their open body posture. Their confidence indicates that they can carry both their own heart and that of their love.

❧

Āyurveda clearly diagnoses the craving for sex as a state of aggravated *pitta*. Especially when the person is craving the act and not the person with whom to engage, Āyurveda reminds us we are isolating the action from its purpose, driving the car without knowing where we are going.

In such cases, we should engage in *pitta*-pacifying activities to lower the imbalance, allowing our natural state of sexuality to flourish. Time in nature, eating sweet, fresh-made, cooling food and cold baths are recommended. One may also put sandalwood paste on the forehead, the fontanelle and the navel. One may drink water that has been put in the moonlight of the full moon or water that has sat overnight in a jar of coriander seeds and rock sugar. Cooling *pranayama*, such as *shitali* and *sitkari* can also provide some relief. *Pitta*-balancing herbs, which must be used only when tailored to a person's body and individual needs, include *amalaki,* cumin, mint, *shatavari, palasha, brahmi* and *aloe*. Over time, the use of these herbs, foods and regimens balances the sex drive, not obliterating it but also not letting it control one's mind and actions.

Discriminative and selective practices, and engagement with conscious intimacy are believed to be the best path to *hita*, best translated as a harmonious and good life. Often mistranslated in English as celibacy, *brahmacharya* does not mean the absence of sexual contact. This translation was probably propagated by the Christian, puritanical influences on Sanskrit translations since the 1750s. *Brahmacharya* is the *charana*, or walk, towards *Brahma*, the Creator, signalling an attitude towards oneness and mental purity. As taught by the masters, *brahmacharya* is the purposeful and wilful engagement in relationships with other humans. There is a choice to engage others on different levels, either only mentally and emotionally (as we do with family members and friends) or in physical proximity (as with housemates and family with which we live) or emotional, physical and spiritual intimacy, as with our sexual–emotional partner.

True *brahmacharya* involves conscious work to understand people who may harm our development by not supporting our mind's growth. If they are selfishly motivated rather than commensal in their activities with us, or if they are not at a similar place of evolution spiritually, we should be careful about the levels at which we engage with them. Engagement in the sexual act for pure physical pleasure, with no attention to breathing exercises and *prana* can lead to disturbances in the body's flows and is discouraged. It aggravates the *dosha*s. Release of energy without re-harnessing through the body's nerve and energy channels depletes *ojas* but is the usual practice for most people engaging in the sexual act. Thus, the rishis discourage it until one learns how to harness that energy of orgasm, one aspect of sacred *tantra*. Once a person learns how to harness the energy, one is exempted from the common guidelines of sex.

Engagement of the senses, in alignment with our body's capacity, is crucial. Harmony with our body in its season and the seasons of nature preserves its vitality. Engagement with people who are able to be intimate requires work to eliminate fear, distrust and deceptive practices that sometimes evolve. It is believed that since society did not have the ability to provide tutorials to each person for evolution of such readiness, en masse it was easier to discourage whimsical intimacy and thus the mistranslation of the term *brahmacharya* continued.

True intimacy with the self integrates soul, mind and body, as well as emotional trust and harmonious mental intimacy with family, friends and teachers, allowing us to lead resilient lives and protecting us from the imbalances that disarm us and lead to disease. It is simple but not easy for most adults.

The following rebalance excess sexual desire:

- Time in nature
- Sweet, fresh-made and cooling food
- Cold baths
- Sandalwood paste on the forehead, the fontanelle and the navel
- Water kept in the moonlight of the full moon or water that has sat overnight in a jar of coriander seeds and rock sugar
- Cooling *pranayama*, such as *shitali* and *sitkari*
- Herbs such as *amalaki,* cumin, mint, *shatavari, palasha, brahmi* and aloe

When intimacy, trust and emotional engagement align with the act of sex, sex becomes powerful and deeply ecstatic.

For years, I have worked actively in the movement to end violence against women and learning about power, violence and the use of sex to propagate hurt.

It started when a close friend in college told me, shaking, one night that she had been raped by a mob of boys, tied up and forced to endure repeated different types of intercourse while the master leader, a senior at a fraternity, commanded this as a dare event, part of the recruitment and hazing process for freshmen at our university. Virgin men could not belong to their fraternity, so he had helped them 'to belong'. Shockingly, 40 per cent women attending university in the US have been molested.

Bewildered and shocked, I watched her grades plummet, her self-control disengage. I watched her seething anger rise after she told her sister and was warned to stay quiet as they were from a known family. Quietly, she disappeared from her potential spot on the stage of history. She later went to medical school and worked as a surgeon, cutting people open and shutting off her tender feelings with the bling of money, a doctor's prestige and a safe shelter.

From her reaction, I felt compelled to complete a training programme in ending violence against women, one of the first in America, called Women Organized Against Rape. I wanted to understand what happened to her and why the act of rape is different from getting mugged or hit by a car. Why does it make women so vulnerable? In the training, I learnt that men and children can also be raped and that the highest number of rape cases occur in the household, between man and wife, and sometimes parent and child. It was a shocking awakening for me and left me wanting to know more about the privacy of sex and why we cannot talk about an act that can destroy a person's mind, just as it can take them to ecstasy.

In most countries, privacy surrounding the sexual relationship is tantamount to sacred ground. No one talks about what happens between two people in an intimate relationship. It is considered a biological need that puts men on vulnerable ground, causing abdications from prestigious positions in society and justifying 'crimes of passion', in which people feel compelled to instil violence in the name of their lover.

From the training, I learnt how to advocate for people who have been bullied and violated and feel despondent, desperate or so vulnerable that they cannot take the courses of action that society offers. In addition, they battle with the enigma of stigma and the double standard that a woman's vagina is so sacred that her virgin status is required to make her pure enough to wed a prince, yet so lacking in sanctity that when she is raped, the crime is given less punishment than when a man's car is stolen. A multitude of problems around consent also arise because sex also has an edge of dominance. What I learnt is that rape is an act of violence, not sex. It uses the sexual organs because these are vulnerable organs through which we wield power; the power to rule a nation by begetting sons and the power to give birth. By condoning sexual violence, we lose our inner power and lose power as a society.

This enigma of privacy around the sexual act prevents proper education about the development of intimacy. Being able to engage in a mature relationship with someone is a learnt skill, which we acquire generally at home and in our first witnessing of relationships between parents, relatives and neighbours. This we adopt as our norm, only adjusting our beliefs once we grow into adults where a larger pool of education can provide us with food for thought on how we will behave. But society is filled with mixed messages, giving little counselling on how to be intimate with one's own soul so that it can connect to another and then use that connection as a basis for physical intimacy.

Add to this a confusing mix of complicated cultural norms surrounding marriage, love and sexual practices, and one has no instructions on how to behave unless successful family and friends can teach. And even there lies a complication because family and friends cannot instruct a person how to behave intimately, how to allure, where to touch, where to kiss and how to press.

Kautilya and Vatsayana solved this problem by creating a user's manual at a time when Buddhism had swept the land and more men were finding God than finding a partner. The world-famous Kama Sutra instructs in detailed prose how to engage with a partner following the spontaneity of desire and also following the rules of society. Without denying the natural tendency for shame,

Vatsayana skillfully arouses the reader while maintaining a didactic tone. While some of the practices are outlawed and illegal in today's society, the book provides a nest of ideas for couples who wish to explore the first two scenes of the sexual act: allure and arousal. The purpose of these books was to re-engage in copulation and child bearing, coupling their interest in spirituality and self-understanding with an investment in relationships and the challenges and rewards of helping children grow.

~ • 38 • ~

Recalling the Day

As often as she could, my mother would come into each of our rooms late at night, after all the guests had left or been put to bed, and all the rooms were clean and closed. In the dark, as it was usually past my bedtime, she would either wake me by sitting at the edge of the bed or call to me from inside the door. As she sat on the bed, we would chat as I sometimes scratched her back or massaged her hands or feet. Sometimes, she would climb under the blanket and sit and talk with me for an hour. We would discuss my school, her woes with her siblings and their antics and issues, or something about my father's work troubles. She would ask about my ever-challenging school issues, as I was perpetually ostracized due to my skin colour, young age, grades or non-endearing, questioning attitude that slowly became combustible as I approached adolescence.

On special days, such as holidays or birthdays, she would recount an earlier year, showering me with blessings for the coming future and reciting spontaneous Sanskrit mantras for invoking the gods. She could make any day special, by remembering anniversaries of our multitude of family members, ancestors, her various journeys through many countries or my father's colourful career. She would begin with a sigh, then recount memories of her father or her mother who had died when she was nineteen, and a story would emerge from the ethers and land in my bedroom, transporting us to Calcutta, Kashi or Jessore of an earlier decade.

Sometimes she would recall the day itself, informing me of events and news of which my school-going life was unaware. She would warn us of coming days, journeys my father planned and relatives who were planning to visit or plant themselves as 'guests' for a few months. Some of the guests were highly anticipated, and I rejoiced with the advance notice, planning handmade gifts and food preparations for their arrival. Together, my mother and I discussed unresolvable problems between my sisters. Often, we discussed my forays into ambition, as I dreamed with her of what I wanted to do with my life and how I resented society for controlling my flight. She liked my room because I never slept with it untidy. I wanted to wake up to perfection, so I always set things to be visually clean before the lights went out. My mother would comment that my room was like a museum, and we would laugh. Then she, satisfied with her massage, would rise and bid me to finish my prayers and sleep.

The evening is the best time for planning the next day's activities, food and errands. Of course, unpredictable things can happen the next day, but a loosely planned day helps get things done and spend time doing good for ourselves, our families and others.

Many tools have been developed to help us get organized: daily planners, bulletin boards, to-do lists, sticky pads, e-calendars, phone reminders and email alerts. The main tool however is will power. Without being compulsive and neurotic about the tasks, it is a great practice to put some order into a coming new day.

One effective method that combines order with gratitude is to end each day with time in a daily diary. Looking to the page for that day, I write three things that I accomplished that day and three things that I am grateful for. On the following page, I list three things that I need to have done the following day; I choose tasks that can be completed without much difficulty. Often, I include one step of a larger task and choose that for my list. The following evening, as I sit to summarize what I have accomplished, I see whether I have accomplished the three tasks I proposed to do. Over time, the three tasks become a guide for my mind to affirm to my body that I can do what I set out to do. Of course, there are days when the unpredictable dominates and I come home grateful to have survived the tumult. Even on those days, my list of gratitude is long.

~ • 39 • ~

Meditation and Night-time Yoga

Before bed each night, my father would visit the altar room. He would switch on the light, utter some sounds and then move to his bedroom. My mother did the same. It did not matter that we lived in a Christian environment, or that they were tired. It did not matter whether others took the time to visit the altar room or not, though they would urge us to visit before going to sleep. It was a personal journey into that room, meant for them and their wishes at the feet of God.

My mother sits for some minutes, moving into asanas and delving into silence. As we discuss the impending dismantling of the room, she quietly tells me that in this room she prayed for each of us to go to college, which she had to quit during her first semester when her father died. She deeply wanted to be a formally educated woman, but saddled with four children, a zoo of siblings and nephews and my father, she gave up her dreams and turned them to the *seva* of others. She confides that in this room she prays that her children will reach their potential, lifted by the hands of the Divine, who should touch them in a way they did not touch her. As we enter this altar room for these last few days, she smiles and then retires to their bedroom, knowing that each of her girls has completed college and is healthy and financially independent. For a woman who has survived more than a few homes broken by wars and the partition of Bengal, my mother's prayers have potentiated this room and created the magic of our family's life.

Even now, as my father hobbles upstairs with his cane and broken body, betrayed by God from doing all he had wished to do, he turns the corner towards their bedroom, stops at the altar room, opens the door and pauses. I will never know whether he does the same mantras or whether he can still think the same way he did when I used to watch him during my childhood. I do not know whether this stop has just become a meaningless ritual, but I do know that if we ever try to take down the pictures from the walls or change the altar room, my father does not like it. It will have to be the last room we dismount as we pack up the house. It will be the last disconnection from the palace he created.

Each night before bed, a quiet period is a must. Rather than turning on the television to watch the horrors of nightly shows or what occurred that day on the news, or the modern antics of journalism and advertising, one should spend time in quiet. The computer and the radio should be turned off. A quick night-time meditative walk in the moonlight during the warm months can be a way to invoke the quiet. During the cold or wet seasons, a cup of herbal tisane and a delightful book can precede the wind down, but there should be a time for quiet breathing exercises, contemplation and emptiness of the mind. Soft, slow stretching yoga poses on a clean floor or on the bed with deep, gentle breathing exercises should be done. The Chandra Namaskar is the day's counterpart for a complete series, but a practice specific to each individual is perfect. A quiet candle can aid meditation, dimming lights and allowing the inner mind to awaken as the senses are less stimulated. This is a time for the self even if you are in the company of others in your bedroom.

These days, many people feel uncomfortable in such quiet. They reflexively keep the television, radio or computer playing until they fall asleep. But this does not calm the *vāta*. To move towards silence, begin by turning off all electronics. Read a book or write in your journal. After that is comfortable, light a candle and put away all books and reading. Become aware of turning off the senses. Move into a quiet state over time, where meditation and quiet become so delicious that they are the preferred activity before bed.

- Evolve a schedule to wind down the day.
- Practise breathing exercises, stretching yoga poses, a night-time walk, reading, writing in your journal or meditation before falling asleep.
- Avoid disturbing films, news or reading just before bed.
- Agree with your bed partner that all arguments and strife will be discussed in the light of day, not at the end of it.

~ • 40 • ~

Getting to Bed on Time

As tiny tots, my mother spent the early evening preparing us for a 7 p.m. bedtime. Over the years, after the first two children, the move to America and the television in the living room, she became more lenient. My youngest sister would often stay awake until 10 p.m., watching television laying atop my father's chest until he would lift her and put her to bed. My older sister and I were conditioned by that time however, and we would finish our homework and trot off happily to bed, enticed by the lull of slumber.

During college, there was no way to get to bed by 9 or 10 p.m. It was only at midnight that the library closed. In the dormitory, pizzas would arrive in the wee hours, and parties would begin at 1 a.m. To stay in tune with classmates and friends, who were scattered all over campus all day, one had to stay awake at night to connect, chat and work together on last-minute homework. Sometimes, a nap in the library or an early evening nap was required, but otherwise the zing of a cup of coffee and the excited, electric atmosphere of the college hallways kept us awake. Parents and family would call in the evening. One year, my roommate joined the crew and had to awaken at 5 a.m. each morning for her workout and rowing practice on the Schulkyll River. Due to her, we got to bed by 11 p.m. for a few months.

Schedules in graduate school, medical school and residency were worse. We were regularly given work that stretched into the midnight hours, either drug doses to laboratory animals or petri dishes every 4–6 hours, or coveted microscope time, which was hard to get during the day. During the years on call in the hospital, there was no alignment with the hours of the day. We floated from emergency to emergency, exam to exam. There were no other necessary time points.

As the old house now yawns its readiness to sleep, my father calls me to him to turn out the light. He quietly recalls the story of the first night we arrived in this house, how we were all too excited to sleep and how we had run around getting lost in the maze of rooms. There had been no furniture on that September night. We had all slept in a huddle in the dining room with its luscious soft carpet, dozing off near each other, twenty years younger. My mother enters as he is hobbling through words. She finishes his sentences for him and climbs into bed as I sit on the edge of their bed. I smirk, then jump lightly again and again, and ask them, '*Ghummocho, ghummocho*? Are you sleeping?'

❧

Evening rituals should end the day with contemplation, gratitude, awareness and preparation, giving us tasks to adjust ourselves if travelling, making us aware of the environment for the hours of night, when our visual senses are less strong. Āyurveda advises judicious choices in the use of alcohol and engagement in sex when we are tired or unable to discern perceptively. It advises evening meditation practice, conscious recall and review of the day and then the *rasayana* of deep sleep, or *nidra yoga*.

The reality of modern, urban life for many people includes difficulty waking up early. Yet, it is easy for others. Why?

Āyurveda tells us that if our bodies are laden with residues and toxins (*āma*), its natural ability to rise with the sun will be hampered. Just as the sun cannot be seen on a cloudy morning, we cannot find our fire when we are clouded by toxins. Waking after 7 a.m. is a sign that your body has excess toxins. Use this signal to cleanse yourself.

Healthy children over the age of four wake up annoyingly early and energized to start the day of exploring and learning. If they do not wake up bright-eyed, it should be a signal to parents that some intervention may be needed. A child should not be so far from its natural rhythms that it needs to sleep so long. With today's trends towards medicating children from infancy, we see that children tend to sleep longer and feel groggy.

Āyurveda counsels that prolonged harbouring of these toxins creates ageing. The body is not light and free, and tries to push aside toxins it cannot excrete when channels are clogged chronically. It stows the toxins in the walls of the arteries, in crevices around organs, but eventually, frustrated, it begins to shove the toxins into cells. This is the cellular process of ageing. As the body forgets where it stored all the toxins, it becomes harder to cleanse and purify. The same applies to your house and belongings. If you store so much that you cannot remember what you own, the unused items pile up and become burdens. Abundance is the ability to let go and let flow; how much you have is measured by how much you can release into the universe. While the energy is still fresh, use it. Do not let it pile up into fat and fibrosis.

To prepare to wake up early, several routines must be in place. Start with the early morning routine and ensure that all components for completing the routine are organized and ready in the bathroom or toilet case. Next, outline some project or task you want to or need to do. Plan the next steps so that you can implement them when you rise. Have a warm blanket waiting during the cold season or a favourite cup ready for morning tea in the spring. Arrange for a cool, cleansing bath and put on fresh light clothes on a summer morning to start the day. If you tend to be hungry early in the morning, have arrangements for morning food preparations planned. Whether it means a walk to the morning market or walking into the kitchen or your mess hall, mentally planning the routine helps you feed your early morning fire happily. If you tend to be groggy, use music or light a candle or incense to awaken yourself. Have something ready that will lure you into the waking world.

- Waking after 7 a.m. is an indication that the body contains excess toxins. Try to go to bed earlier.
- Plan your mornings the night before.
- Make sure that all the components required to carry out the early-morning routine are in place before you go to bed.
- Have a cold bath and wear fresh clothes to bed in summer.
- Drink a cup of warm milk before bed in the winter, chamomile tea before bed in spring or autumn and a cool glass of water in summer.
- If you tend to be groggy in the morning, prepare music or a candle or incense to help yourself awaken

Modern medicine is also changing its views on the perfect amount of sleep, as emerging science validates new findings and retracts old ones regularly. Several studies, one surveying more than one million adults and another surveying only women, found that people who live the longest reported sleeping for 6–7 hours each night. Studies consistently show that sleeping more than 8 hours a day has been associated with increased risk of dying, possibly because it points to reasons why people will sleep more, such as depression, frustrated socioeconomic status or chronic illness.

On the other side, studies suggest a correlation between lower sleep hours and reduced morbidity only when those who wake after less sleep wake naturally, rather than those who use an alarm or are chronically sleep deprived. Āyurveda tells us to rest well, then lift ourselves out from the suppressed state of too much sleep and find reasons to live.

Āyurveda does not advise 8 hours of sleep for everyone. It never has; it states that people need different amounts of sleep depending on their constitution, the amount of functional digestive fire they have, the amount of toxins they have in their system, their stage of life, the climate and the season. People with more toxins require more time for sleep, as do people with less digestive fire and children in their *kapha* stage of life.

Begin by mentally asking yourself to harmonize with the natural rhythms of the natural environment. Keep a log of daily rhythms, monitoring your hunger, purges and sleep. Set goals to go to bed earlier each night, adjusting slowly so that your lifestyle and family are not troubled. Keep track of the mornings you more energy or less energy, and the notable events of your days that affect your physical, mental and emotional energy levels. Note when you awaken each morning and when you go to bed. You may notice that you do well with 4–9 hours or anything in between. Sleep is considered to be adequate when there is no daytime sleepiness or dysfunction, and you feel refreshed when you arise. Once you find your own rhythm, stick to it for a month and notice how you feel.

- Keep track of the times when you awaken and when you fall asleep.
- Everyone's requires a different amount of sleep; it could be anywhere between 4 and 9 hours.

To invoke the power of rising early, determine the time of sunrise in your area to capitalize on the *vāta* hours of the morning.

The last challenge of optimizing the *vāta* period and Āyurvedic guidelines for *Brahma muhurta* is finding what activities you want to do with the extra time of the early morning. For many people, extra projects await. But this is not a time for adding more work to the day; it is a time of investment in spirit, self and security. While this is difficult for people who are less emotionally connected or mentally mature, it is an important time that teaches us the lessons of life that no one else can. The best options for activity are to find something with the theme of meditation, spiritual study, yoga or time in nature.

To start yourself waking early, begin by aiming to wake up 15 minutes earlier and having a cup of hot water after you awaken. Keep waking earlier till you rise at 7 a.m. and give yourself time to see the morning and appreciate it. Then continue waking fifteen minutes earlier until you reach the span of time that is *Brahma muhurta*. Watch how your mind and body feel. If your schedule is completely unable to adjust to this, and you waken late each day, attempt a realistic goal of setting an alarm to awaken at 5 a.m., stay awake for 20–30 minutes, then go back to bed and sleep until you are rested or have to waken for work or life obligations. In most regions, the ideal time to awaken is between 5.30 and 7 a.m., depending on the time of year and the latitude. See how it feels to awaken and greet the sun and how it connects you with the awesome forces of nature.

~ • 41 • ~

Rasayana: Vitality and the Raising of Agni

I often ponder what did take its toll on my father's *agni*, the day he suffered a stroke from which he has not yet recovered. During medical school, I rushed 750 miles to his hospital bedside as he moved his left limbs for the last time. I learnt every detail of his case and discussed all the medical options for him. I reviewed his CT scans with their large series of holes in the prefrontal cortex, and I reviewed his blood tests. When I saw the way he was treated in the academic hospital in the second week of July that year, I realized that my faith in the modern medical education system was interrupted. The ICU staff lacked the ability to see him as a human, and their fixation on his individual laboratory test numbers was scary. Their determination that his future should align with their predictions was disheartening. Because he lost his ability to speak English, they determined that all his foreign languages were 'mumblings' and denied him rehabilitation.

Since that week, I have spent nights combing through neuroscience textbooks, trying to decipher what happened in his brain to cause his stroke, what doctors wrote off by calling it a MCA (middle cerebral artery) ischemic episode. I have searched for ways to look beyond those predictions because they are, frankly, wrong and limited by the vista that modern medicine takes. My father lost so much of his function, and yet he recovered the ability to speak small sentences, walk, understand the news, eat, dress himself and enjoy music. And he holds tight to his *dinacharya*, the morning routine, as though it defines him and his right to heal.

I wonder what he sees when he looks in the mirror. He seems to have an excellent memory and recalls the most amazing details from random prompts in our conversations, the television, a book or an old item taken from a drawer or closet. Does he see the determination and the drive to live, or does he see the disappointments and stunning failure of losing one's body to a stroke? His genius is slowly being consumed by periodic falls, blood tests that precede aborted attempts to start aggressive new drugs from aggressive new doctors and loneliness trapped in the world of the disabled.

What I remember is the FDA raided our home and his basement laboratory that day, just before the stroke came to take him hostage. They suspected he was involved in nefarious activities, daring to explore science, writing papers and creating evidence without a university affiliation, an NIH grant or the accolades of the men who sell themselves to science. He had chosen to explore the cow and that had led him unbridled to new vistas, making new discoveries that pharmaceutical executives had threatened to suppress and grant makers had discouraged.

His life is my lesson. Because of him, I am packing this house and we are all leaving. Because he did not tend to his *agni* and his *dosha*s, things got severely out of balance, and he lost himself in his passion and ambition. Each of us is to blame when we do not take care of our mind and our body. Each of us has the responsibility to keep the boat steady, the fire burning and the car on course on the highway of life. Through periodic fits of tears and anger, as I pack and fill boxes incessantly, a lotus petal opens as my heart effuses with compassion for this man who is my father. His failure to care for his body, like the failures of most of my patients, is my lesson to learn what is true, what heals, what medicine truly is and to share it with my students and patients.

bibhēti-durbalō'bhīkṣṇaṁ-dhyāyati-vyathitēndriyaḥ |
duśchāyō-durmanā-rūkṣaḥ-kṣāmaścaivaujasaḥ-kṣayē ||*73*||
hṛdi-tiṣṭhati-yacchuddhaṁ-raktamīṣatsapītakam |
ōjaḥ-śarīrē-saṅkhyātaṁ-tannāśānnā-vinaśyati ||*74*||

The decline of *ojas* (resilience and vitality) begins with living in fear, constant weakness and lack of fortification with food and happiness, worry, affliction of pain via the sense organs, loss of complexion, hopelessness and lack of cheer, roughness and emaciation. That which dwells in the heart, white, yellow and reddish in colour, is known as the *ojas* of the body. If it is destroyed, the person will also perish.

Caraka Samhita,
Sūtra-sthāna; chapter 17, slokas 73–74

Āyurveda tells us that the purpose of our daily routine is to keep us healthy, to build our fire and give us the energy, power and focus to do what we are here in this life to do. When the transformative properties of the body are balanced and transmuting matter and energy back and forth as needed, there exudes an inner radiance, a subtle energy of fire, primal vigour, radiance of vitality and an unfolding of all higher perceptual capacities, called *ojas*. The person shows courage, perception and insight. In the mind and consciousness, there is a force propelling the mind and allowing it to perceive and determine; digest impressions, ideas, emotions, accumulated insight and vitality of our spiritual aspiration; and to light the soul.

The game of fire requires us to live in cycles, since the earth also lives in cycles. There are cycles in nature waiting to guide you. The way to know how to change, what to change and when to shift requires a pivoting point. That pivot is your internal digestive fire.

When your fire is low, all the routines of the day should focus on nurturing the fire, kindling it and helping it grow. Rest, light food, fasting, exercise, sex, cold baths and certain herbs will kindle the fire. When the fire is high, all the routines of the day should focus on keeping the fire centered in the gut so that it will not spread or burn out, as it will have the tendency to move just as fire moves. Focussed work, good sleep only for the needed time, clean pure food, meals on time, sufficient movement and exercise, cold baths and certain herbs will keep the fire strong, warm and transformative.

When people want to change their lives, they wonder how a few routines can do it, when most of their hours are spent in a world dominated by other people's priorities. The key to *dinacharya* is to set up the body, mind, senses and soul in the beginning and end of the day, cleaning the senses and kindling the fire, so that whatever is put into it will be cooked to the body's satisfaction and will improve the mind and benefit the soul.

What draws healers to Āyurveda is its theories that hold true when they are tested in the real world. Routines, treatments and herbs, when used according to the Āyurvedic theories of *dosha*, *dhatu*, *srotas*, āma and agni really work. The key is to learn enough authentic Āyurveda so that you can experiment perceptively on yourself, your friends and your family. Then, after some level of exploration, you must delve into the original works, in Sanskrit, to really internalize and digest the depth and meaning of Āyurveda for your own life. It is a tall task for some, but Sanskrit will increase your fire and will revitalize your *agni* as the sounds and concepts connect your mind to your senses and your soul.

I have found that learning Āyurveda has raised my *ojas* and revitalized my *agni*. Moreover, my students and patients that take on learning Āyurveda have been rewarded with the greatest gift of all: health.

❧

~ • 42 • ~

Sleep

My mother is going to sleep in, she says, exhausted from her forced labour as the twenty- four hour caretaker of the man who lifted her on his wings and flew her to Europe and America. She is now trapped with her eagle, ever devout but growing tired of the recurrent traumas of his falls as a paralysed man. She used to rise without fail at about 4 a.m. for years. Now, it is time to let her rest. The ordeal of my father's condition, as long as it lasts, is beginning to take its toll on her, and she needs extra rest.

As the day ends, I take over the task of checking the house and to check that all the doors are closed and all the windows secure. I travel through the house, recounting memories of all I have learnt, all I have witnessed and all I have loved about this house. My routines have been tested and refined in this house, with the guidance of my mother and father and all the visitors, relatives and friends who have traversed it.

It is time to sleep. I know that tonight I will need a little extra sleep, as my day has been filled with memories of sadness and deep contemplation as I packed the house. I am still reminiscing as I enter into my night routine, first to boil some water, transfer it to the copper vessel in the oven and take a few sips of clean water only if I need to quench any thirst. Next, I visit the bathroom and tie my hair, rinse my face with water, rinse my mouth, apply some tooth powder and brush. I rinse my mouth again and inspect my tongue. I pat my face dry using upward strokes. Next, I apply some ghee to my eyes using outward horizontal motions and grind some sandalwood paste for my face, applying it outward and in the direction of the facial hair. I wash my feet and head into the bedroom shoeless, where I undress into light, clean nightclothes and hang my day clothing on the chair to air out from the day. I pull out my *asana* mat and do a few yoga poses, stretching as I monitor what my body is saying. I say a couple of mantras and move onto my bed, where I sit for a moment to recount the day, fill my heart consciously with gratitude, check the time and then lie down to sleep, usually either on a hard mat or on the floor. This routine itself has become itself a conditioning, and I notice that I am called towards sleep as my body moves through the motions. I am grateful that I do not have insomnia or the inability to settle down most nights. And soon, I sleep.

While the rules for sleep state 'early to bed and early to rise', they apply to the healthy, strong and those who are not mentally distressed. Extra pain and strain beyond what a person can bear will cause her to require more sleep. Āyurveda says each person is different, with different capacities for bearing suffering and upset. Shocks require extra time to heal and extra sleep. Pregnant women, children and people convalescing will need extra sleep. People with extra *kapha* will be predisposed to stagnancy and stillness. People with excess *āma* will also want more sleep, but because it is a pathological condition, it will be better for them to resist the temptation and work to wake early.

Another set of rules involves how to set up the bed space for good sleep, called sleep hygiene. The bedroom should be kept as a still, sacred space if possible. A smaller room with simple, clean visual lines and rest-promoting furnishings is ideal. Electric wires near the bed are not advised, as electric current creates electromagnetic fields, which will have subtle effects on your own electromagnetic field. Electronic equipment, especially wi-fi, is therefore, not advised. There is a high concentration of positive ions emitted from electronic appliances, so a great bedroom will be free of these. Clutter on the whole should be eliminated from the bedroom. The bed should have the head facing east or south and never north, as the polarity of the earth should not be aligned with the spinal fluid and its subtle pulses, called craniosacral pulsation.

Āyurveda says a hard bed is best rather than a cushy mattress or air cushion, waterbed or soft surface. Physiologically, this is because the muscles and bones maintain their strength and solidity as a result of resistance. Astronauts lose their bone density and muscle mass precipitously due to distance from gravity for long periods of time. When the body sleeps on a soft mattress for 6–8 hours each night, one-third of one's life, the bones do not get resistance against gravity. Instead, sleeping on a hard mat or futon forces the body to condition itself in relation to the other structures with which it is aligned. The spine creates strength within itself to maintain its natural curvature, and the hardness prevents the spine from sagging in response to untoned muscles. A pillow under the neck may be needed until you become accustomed to the hardness.

Āyurveda also advises that you only drink water before bed if you feel truly thirsty. Why provoke your kidneys and make your gut expend extra energy to convert the water into usable energy if it is not needed? It advises you to not eat food less than 3 hours before you sleep, as your *pitta* fire will be busy processing your gut and not your mind. Do some stretching or some yoga or take an evening walk to help you get some circulation before settling down for the night.

The room where you sleep should have a pleasant, restful ambience. A candle, some *agarbatti* of a light fragrance or some flowers will enhance a mood for quiet. Clean sheets should be on the bed, both on top of the surface, as well as between you and any blankets you use. Pillow covers and casings should be changed 1–2 times a week, depending on how clean your hair is and whether you sleep with your mouth open. You should not share your pillow with another person, as the exudates from their orifices may fall on the pillow during sleep.

The room should be dark where you sleep, to help your pineal gland know the dark zone. When your brain can sense stark contrast between dark and light, it produces clearer signals for hormones. Dark curtains are therefore advised, especially if your room overlooks a light post or in the city.

The bedroom is a safe space, where a person can safely place his/her body while the mind and spirit escape to the land of sleep. Ensure that your bedroom door can be closed if needed. Set policies in the house if interruption is likely to occur regularly. If you have a bedmate, ensure that the bed is a no war zone, setting boundaries together that arguments or strong discussions or emotional tugs needed to be hoisted to another room and not continued in the bedroom. Use the bedroom only for sleep and for intimacy, closeness and loving, where good-hearted, strong support is abundant, not negative emotions. Do not allow food on the bed. Do not smoke in bed. Do not use it as an entertainment zone. It should not be covered with excess pillows, accessories or clothes, papers or books. Keep a clean bed, making the bed every morning after lifting the sheet and brushing it off. Change the sheet if a lot of activity has occurred or if the sheet is not clean.

Once you have established a sacred zone for sleeping, prepare yourself with a night routine that includes emptying your bladder, changing into clean nightclothes made of natural fabrics such as cotton or silk, and washing your feet.

With these guidelines, do a self-study on your own sleep needs and know how much sleep you need. Remember the guideline that an hour of sleep before midnight is worth 2 hours of sleep after midnight. If you want it, a good routine will evolve for you until you find that you are sleeping optimally. This will be such a blessing that you will realize the importance of good sleep hygiene.

Just before you sleep, sit quietly and say a small prayer. Thank yourself for your day, no matter how challenging it was. You lived the day and you have the choice of how to live tomorrow.

In my dreams, I often return to the forest of my childhood, the village where my ancestors lived many years before the trees were ripped down. I go there because the knowledge of nature and its forces are there. My subtle self knows that I will heal when I am submerged in its forces. It takes me there to play, to dream and to grow. I breathe deep, healing, plentiful clean air, and I am permitted to be all that I am, unapologetically sensual and daringly spiritual. Here, Āyurveda is alive, not through books or writings, but through the knowledge that lives deeply within the plants and the way they live together harmoniously in their ecosystem, ready to teach anyone who will sit silently and listen to them. Each moment in nature can remind us to follow a sequence and walk forward, aligning us with the forces of the day until we can analyse the science and validate what nature has been trying to teach us all along.

Epilogue

When we find our calling in life, we become anchored to our souls. The search for paths to true healing and the right to walk those paths is my calling. During my active practice of mainstream medicine, I found neither balance nor health. When I integrated conventional medicine with Āyurveda, things came alive. To make Āyurveda more accessible to my students, patients, friends and colleagues in New York, my medical practice 'Good Medicine Works' anchored the observation of *dosha*, *dhatu*, *guna* and the soul in every prescription. My patients loved the approach, and slowly, the practice gained the reputation for healing conditions uncured by modern medicine. This book took birth.

Intense immersion became a necessity. In allegiance to the authentic wisdom of the Āyurveda forefathers, a hunger developed to work deeper toward understanding disease and self-care, to study *ojas*. Not hiding from the original Sanskrit was the only way to proceed into the ocean of wisdom. It has clarified many ideas about physiology and biochemistry by seeing the ecosystem of the body in its various environments.

As I finish this book sitting in Banaras Hindu University, re-submerging myself into PhD studies, I am ever grateful to the many learned clinician-scholars of Āyurveda throughout India that I have met as a senior Fulbright Scholar this year, who have welcomed me into their circle, advised, inspired and guided my thinking as this book has evolved. I am also grateful to my patients who showed me that practical realities mean more than scientific theory. Medical science must translate into the real world of life and living if it is to have meaning in the eyes of its users.

The best way to prove the worth of anything is to use it in one's own life. For if one does not trust the methods and practices of Āyurveda when one falls ill, what is the value of the science? I offer this book as my testament that authentic Āyurveda works. During the writing of this book, I used my body as a laboratory, experimenting with each of the forty-two prescriptions and trying to understand the shastras more fully. Perfecting my own daily routine, as I read and studied the shastras, I began to lose weight. From the time I started actively writing until the completion of this book, I have lost 26 kg without dieting and without much effort, keeping one main principle at the centre of it all: how to balance the *agni*. Every decision was centered around that calculation, forcing me to learn what Āyurveda would recommend, adapting that to the modern day as needed and obeying that prescription.

It was only after my father breathed for the last time and his ashes were returned to the Ganga that I could find focus to write this book and return to the land that had taught him and me Āyurveda. I hope you will enjoy the blessing of my parents' wisdom and benefit from it as much as I have. Namashkar.

A Note on the Author

Living between Manhattan and Kashi, Dr Bhaswati Bhattacharya is a licensed, board-certified physician, integrating 'Good Medicine' with Ayurveda for the past fifteen years. She is Clinical Assistant Professor of Family Medicine at Weill Cornell Medical College and a PhD researcher in Āyurveda at Banaras Hindu University. She is a 2014 senior Fulbright–Nehru Scholar, recipient of American Medical Association's Leadership Award and the first Indian to speak at Commencement Exercises at Harvard University. Her work is featured in the documentary, *Healers: Journey into Āyurveda, on The Discovery Channel*. Her website is: www.drbhaswati.com.